Is There No Place on Earth for Me?

Books by Susan Sheehan

Ten Vietnamese
A Welfare Mother
A Prison and a Prisoner
Is There No Place on Earth for Me?

Is There No Place on Earth for Me?

Susan Sheehan

FOREWORD by
ROBERT M. COLES, M.D., Ph.D.

HOUGHTON MIFFLIN COMPANY BOSTON
1982

Most of the contents of this book originally appeared, in slightly different form, in *The New Yorker*. The Foreword by Robert M. Coles and the Afterword by Susan Sheehan are published here for the first time.

Library of Congress Cataloging in Publication Data

Sheehan, Susan.
Is there no place on earth for me?

Originally appeared, in slightly different form, in the New Yorker.
1. Schizophrenics — United States — Biography.
2. Frumkin, Sylvia. 3. Creedmoor Psychiatric Center.
I. Title.
RC514.S49 616.89'82'0924 [B] 81-20245
ISBN 0-395-31871-8 AACR2

Printed in the United States of America

D 10 9 8 7 6 5 4 3 2 1

For Maria Gregory Sheehan

Acknowledgments

I am gratefully in debt to Dr. William L. Werner, the Director of Creedmoor Psychiatric Center, who welcomed me to Creedmoor one day in April 1978, and who encouraged me to spend twenty-four hours a day at his institution. "Talk to everyone, go to all our meetings, and let the public know how bad things are here, and perhaps they will get better," he said. Dr. Werner died suddenly in September 1978, but fortunately his open-door policy was continued by his successors. Hundreds of patients and staff members helped me during the three years I spent researching and writing this book. It is not possible to publish the names of any of the patients, and to thank several hundred staff members would be to publish a book of lists, so I acknowledge with profound thanks the three people at Creedmoor with whom I worked most closely and who gave so generously of their time and knowledge and kindness: Rita Amatulli, Hermine Plotnick, and the "specialist in psychopharmacology" referred to in the text, whose name is Dr. Gideon Seaman.

It is also a pleasure to have a page on which to thank some of my colleagues at *The New Yorker:* Brendan Gill, Milton Greenstein, Ann Goldstein, Helen Ruttencutter,

Nancy Holyoke, Eleanor Gould, Mary Norris, Edward Stringham, David Jackson, Sharon Lerner, Joseph R. Carroll, John M. Murphy, Bernard J. McAteer, William J. Fitzgerald, John Broderick, Patrick J. Keogh, Luis R. Feliciano, Juan Cruz, Jr., Bruce J. Diones, Peter Deitch, and Carmine J. Graziano, Jr. William Shawn, the editor of *The New Yorker,* is the only editor in the world who would have let a writer try to write about such a sad and difficult subject and who would then have published a hundred thousand words on the subject. No *New Yorker* writer could do better than to have John Bennet as an editor and Martin Baron as a checker to verify all the factual information in *Is There No Place on Earth for Me?*

I am also thankful to the Ford Foundation for its generous financial assistance; to Jane and Andrea Goldwyn and Harvey Pincus; to the Research Facilities Office of the Library of Congress; and to Austin Olney, Nan A. Talese, Gail Ross, and Clay Morgan of Houghton Mifflin.

Most of all I thank Sylvia Frumkin, her parents, and her sister for signing the consent forms required for this book, and for welcoming me into their lives so that I could tell their story. As a result of the Frumkins' cooperation, I had access to Sylvia Frumkin's psychiatric records and I was able to do almost all of my reporting at first hand. I was on the ward taking shorthand notes of Miss Frumkin's monologues. I was at the Frumkins' dinner table on the Jewish New Year. I was sleeping in the bed next to Sylvia Frumkin's at the Creedmoor hotel the snowy night she decided to run away.

The names of almost all the patients in this book, including Sylvia Frumkin, have been changed, as have the names of most Creedmoor personnel, and some details have been altered to disguise their identities.

Contents

Foreword

by Robert M. Coles, M.D., Ph.D.

"Is there no place on earth for me?" has been asked by countless men and women who have never seen a psychiatrist or spent time in a mental hospital. Children the world over quite commonly ask themselves and their parents terribly provocative and haunting questions — questions that are certainly "existentialist," in that they are aimed at comprehending life's mysteries. After a while, though, many of us give up and immerse ourselves in the ebb and flow of a particular existence. It is left to our writers and our artists, not to mention our scientists, to keep alive the intense curiosity, the disarming awe, the unashamed and driven wonder that so often characterize nursery-school children as they pester and plead for answers. Gauguin's powerful painting *Where do we come from? What are we? Where are we going?* was finished in 1897, just before the aging artist, shut off and fearful, ailing physically and low in spirits, attempted (in an act of desperation) to kill himself by taking arsenic. His paintings showed, nevertheless, how alive he was, how attentive still to the kind of moral and psychological inquiry it is in our nature to make.

Most of us are not granted the genius of a Gauguin, or of, say, a philosophical novelist or a metaphysical poet —

the genius of men and women who transform their questions into inspired canvases or words. But even those of us with the least intellectual or artistic inclinations can still, by virtue of our humanity, ask the most thoughtful questions. Nor does craziness destroy that capacity; indeed, many men and women wrestle with the meaning of things even while they spend years struggling with terrible fears, with haunting doubts, with delusions and hallucinations that won't go away despite the assurances of doctors and the pills and electric shocks that doctors prescribe.

When I was a psychiatric resident, a patient of mine, a janitor, told me: "I've no education, and I'm loony. I know it, but I still stop and look around and try to figure out what's happening to me, and to these crazy doctors who take care of us crazy patients. I'm not a dog, a rat — not yet!" The downward slope of his mental life was such that, upon occasion, he was convinced that a long dead puppy dog, a childhood acquaintance, lived inside his mind and craved expression — hence the abrupt, mournful barks we who attended him would sometimes hear. At other times, however, we saw a man's searching, reflective mind at work, now and then exerting itself more strenuously than might have been the case had he not been plagued by demons within. One can say this without romanticizing madness as some have done in recent years, without falsely proclaiming it a royal road to truth and wisdom.

Readers of *The New Yorker* met Sylvia Frumkin in the spring of 1981, and readers of this book will soon enough get to know her extraordinarily well, because of a particular writer's observational and literary gifts. Miss Frumkin turns out to be an extremely troubled person whose mind doesn't work, in certain respects, the way most other minds work. The labels psychiatrists use to set Miss Frumkin apart, the diagnostic classifications applied to her, are merely matters of medical convenience — or should be. We don't learn all that much about a patient when we are told that she is "schizophrenic," but we do learn that certain aspects of her mental life are predictably exceptional. Most of us don't hear strange voices commanding us to do this or that. We don't see things that aren't physically there while awake. We don't invent words and use them insistently, provocatively, to the consternation of our neighbors. We don't scream and shout and mumble over and over again for reasons no one can figure out. We don't talk in such a way that even our friends and relatives can't possibly ascertain what in the world we are saying, or mean to say. But Miss Frumkin and thousands upon thousands of other Americans, and millions the world over, have it as their lot to think and feel and behave in such a manner. Yet as we get to know Miss Frumkin we also see her as — what? A seeker, a pilgrim. A person struggling earnestly and honestly with important moral issues. A shrewd observer of her fellow human creatures, no matter how wrong-headed her conclusions about them may be. It is a tribute to Susan Sheehan that her "subject" does not come across as yet another exhibit in the growing literary landscape of American grotesquerie.

No one knows how it comes about that a Sylvia Frumkin has the kind of life we find chronicled in this book. Genes matter, some scientists say. Family life is important, others insist. Early childhood experiences count heavily, a number of doctors emphasize. But there is still plenty of room, one suspects, for speculation and research; room even for words such as *luck, chance, destiny.* Why, one wonders, this person and not that one? I have heard schizophrenic men and women ask that question in the resigned fashion of the Greek tragedians. It is clear that many who seem to have everything against them genetically and environmentally seem to come out reasonably well psychologically, while others, with everything seemingly going in their favor, end up with exceedingly vulnerable, even fragile minds.

It is little consolation, surely, to Miss Frumkin and her parents to know that she is by no means alone in her search for a world in which she can feel understood and accepted. She speaks strange thoughts. She behaves oddly. If many of us scratch our heads and dismiss her as peculiar, as unbalanced, as worthy of confinement, we will soon enough meet one, then another person who is similarly afflicted. In the New Testament (Mark 5) we find Christ contending not just with a certain individual's demonic behavior, but a widespread presence: "My name is Legion: for we are many." Psychiatrists can't emulate the Lord, who rid the Gadarenes of turmoil by removing the "devils" within a substantial number of them (an estimated two thousand!) and lodged them in "a great herd of swine," which promptly "ran violently down a steep place into the sea" — there, of course, to drown. But, in the tradition of the person who described himself as Legion, psychiatrists are able to count, to make an estimate of the quantitative nature of a particular problem. In the *Archives of General Psychiatry* of June 1978, a report from the National Institute of Mental Health tells us that by "conservative" estimate "at least 10 percent of the total population is affected by a mental disorder at any one point in time." In a careful study done in Manhattan during the 1950s, it was found that no less than 23 percent of the adult population "were affected by serious psychiatric impairments at any one point in time." In 1975, the NIMH report declares, approximately thirty million persons were struggling with one or another serious psychiatric difficulty. Well over six million of these troubled individuals received "treatment" in one form or another, and "approximately 1.5 million persons . . . were actually hospitalized."

The issue, then, is clearly the pain and confusion felt by millions of Sylvia Frumkins. It is the aimlessness, melancholy, want of confidence, irresolution, misgivings of all sorts, alarm, terror, and moments of outright panic that torment them. In these pages, an exceptionally able and tenacious observer, willing to work hard and long to achieve the best kind of factual writing, has given us a tactful and scrupulously accurate presentation of this sad and continuing affliction. The dramatic and humorous side of Miss Frumkin's emotional and intellectual life holds our attention and moderates — a bit — our sadness; moreover, she touches us enough to make us look a little more closely at our own assumptions, our moments of stupidity, insensitivity, and prejudice. On the whole, though, we are grateful for being spared a life of hell on earth, and we are grateful, too, for the subtle and penetrating education Susan Sheehan has offered us.

Harvard University
Cambridge, Massachusetts

I

Creedmoor Psychiatric Center

One

Shortly after midnight on Friday, June 16, 1978, Sylvia Frumkin decided to take a bath. Miss Frumkin, a heavy, ungainly young woman who lived in a two-story yellow brick building in Queens Village, New York, walked from her bedroom on the second floor to the bathroom next door and filled the tub with warm water. A few days earlier, she had had her hair cut and shaped in a bowl style, which she found especially becoming, and her spirits were high. She washed her brown hair with shampoo and also with red mouthwash. Some years earlier, she had tinted her hair red and had liked the way it looked. She had given up wearing her hair red only because she had found coloring it every six weeks too much of a bother. She imagined that the red mouthwash would somehow be absorbed into her scalp and make her hair red permanently. Miss Frumkin felt so cheerful about her new haircut that she suddenly thought she was Lori Lemaris, the mermaid whom Clark Kent had met in college and had fallen in love with in the old "Superman" comics. She blew bubbles into the water.

After a few minutes of contented frolicking, Miss Frumkin stepped out of the tub. She slipped on the bathroom floor — it was wet from her bubble-blowing and splashing — and cut the back of her head as she fell. The cut began to bleed. She attempted to stop the bleeding by applying pressure to the cut, then wrapped her head in a large towel and walked back to her bedroom. On the dresser was a bottle of expensive perfume that an aunt and uncle had given her in May as a thirtieth-birthday present. She poured the contents of the bottle on her cut, partly because she knew that perfume contained alcohol and that alcohol was an antiseptic (in 1972, Miss Frumkin had completed a ten-month course qualifying her as a medical secretary), and partly because she suddenly thought that she was Jesus Christ and that her bleeding cut was the beginning of a crown of thorns. She also thought that she was Mary Magdalene, who had poured ointment on Christ. Looking back on the incident six months later, Miss Frumkin was exasperated with herself for having wasted the perfume, which the aunt and uncle had bought in Israel, and which she couldn't replace. "It was the one perfume I've ever had that people complimented me on," she said. "So many people told me I smelled nice when I wore it. I'm sorry I wasted it."

Miss Frumkin's head burned when the perfume came in contact with the open cut, and the bleeding subsided but didn't altogether stop. By then, it was after one o'clock. She put on an old nightgown and went downstairs to the office of the building to tell the night supervisor, Dwight Miller, who was on duty from midnight until eight-thirty, what had happened. Miller looked at the cut, told Miss Frumkin to get dressed, and said he would drive her to the emergency room at Long Island Jewish-Hillside Medical Center, a voluntary hospital in New Hyde Park, a short distance away. The cut didn't look bad, and Miss Frumkin appeared calm about it — calmer than Miller thought he would have been if their situations had been reversed — but he knew that any head injury was potentially serious and should be examined by a doctor. In her room, Miss Frumkin put on her underclothes, a pink-and-white print blouse and matching pink-

and-white striped skirt, a pair of brown sandals, a Timex watch she had borrowed from her mother after losing her own watch, a pair of glasses with octagonal frames (Miss Frumkin is very nearsighted), and a beige poncho with colorful designs, which her sister had brought her as a gift from a recent trip to Peru. She took with her a large tan pocketbook that bulged with notebooks, a bankbook, makeup, and other paraphernalia, and walked downstairs.

As Miller started the car, turned on the car radio, and began to drive toward the hospital, Miss Frumkin seemed to get excited. The radio was playing Paul McCartney's song "The Lovely Linda," and he was singing the words "La, la, la, la, la, the lovely Linda." Unknown to Miller, Miss Frumkin thought that McCartney was singing the lyrics sarcastically, because he had fallen in love with her and was no longer in love with Linda, his wife. Miss Frumkin began to talk fervently to the radio. For a time, Miller was afraid she might jump out of the car. Miss Frumkin and Miller arrived at the emergency room of L.I.J.-Hillside at two o'clock. Miss Frumkin was first interviewed and examined by a nurse. For a few minutes, she was in sufficient control of herself to let the nurse take her vital signs, test her neurological responses, and look at her cut, and to answer the questions that the nurse asked. She correctly gave her name and address, an account of her fall, and the names and addresses of her next of kin — her parents, Irving and Harriet Frumkin, who also live in Queens. She became upset while she was waiting to see a doctor and an X-ray technician (she began to speak rapidly, and what she said concerned suffering from hypoglycemia and Wilson's disease and being Cinderella, and didn't make much sense); more upset when the X-ray technician took X rays of her skull and the doctor sewed up the cut (Miss Frumkin was so agitated that the doctor succeeded in putting in only three of five silk sutures he had intended to put in); and still more upset when it turned out that there would be a fairly long wait for the skull X rays to be read. Miss Frumkin got so obstreperous while she and Miller were waiting in the main area of the emergency room that they were shown into one of the small treatment rooms off to one side that the hospital uses to give people privacy, where they were joined by a hospital security guard. Miss Frumkin had made so many difficulties for the doctor who had stitched her cut — by flaunting her medical knowledge, testing his, accusing him of incompetence, calling him names, and threatening to sue him and the hospital — that he had called for the psychiatric resident on duty to examine her. In the small treatment room, Miss Frumkin's conduct became increasingly bizarre. She took off all her clothes, accused Miller of kidnapping her and making sexual advances, and then asked Miller and the security guard to have sexual relations with her, saying she hadn't had sex with a man in five years. The minute the two men would cover Miss Frumkin with a hospital gown, she would disrobe again.

Around three o'clock, Dr. Conrad Aaronson, a psychiatric resident, came to observe and question Miss Frumkin. He spent about an hour with her, asking her to tell him about herself and about what had happened to her that morning. He also tried to talk to her about her past. Dr. Aaronson then put down on an L.I.J.-Hillside consultation form his opinions of Miss Frumkin and his recommendations for what should be done with her. Dr. Aaronson wrote that Miss Frumkin was alert and was "oriented in all three spheres" — she knew who she was, where she was, and what day it was. He found her memory for recent and remote events difficult to assess, because she displayed marked "loosening of associations" (ideas slipping off one track and onto another, completely unrelated one) and "circumstantiality" (getting bogged down in a morass of trivial details that impede communication of a central idea), and also because she was extremely agitated, verbally abusive, and uncooperative. In Dr. Aaronson's opinion, Miss Frumkin's insight and judgment were poor, she was "labile" (that is, subject to rapid changes in mood), and she easily became angry, hostile, and threatening. In addition, some of her ideas were paranoid, and she expressed "delusions of reference," which is to say that she misinterpreted incidents and events in the outside world as having a direct personal reference to her: She told Dr. Aaronson not only that Paul McCartney had sung to her but also that she was going to marry another former Beatle, Ringo Starr. Dr. Aaronson described Miss Frumkin as "acutely psychotic." (A psychosis is defined in one standard psychiatric glossary as "a major mental disorder . . . in which the individual's ability to think, respond emotionally, remember, communicate, interpret reality, and behave appropriately is sufficiently impaired so as to interfere grossly with his capacity to meet the ordinary demands of life.") While Dr. Aaronson was questioning Miss Frumkin, her skull X rays had come back; they were negative. He ruled out the possibility that her psychotic behavior was due to physical damage from her fall. His impression of Miss Frumkin's condition was that it was an acute exacerbation of chronic schizophrenia — one of the most common forms of serious mental illness in the world. Dr. Aaronson found that Miss Frumkin was in no shape to return to her room in Queens Village. He wrote in his report, at 4:15 A.M., "Patient removed all her clothing and began chanting and praying on the floor at the conclusion of the interview . . . Patient is in need of emergency hospitalization as she represents a danger to herself and to others in her present condition."

Miss Frumkin was asked if she would like to be admitted to the psychiatric division of L.I.J.-Hillside. Although she had been a psychiatric patient there on two previous occasions — her most recent stay had lasted from February 6, 1978, to May 9, 1978 — and thought highly of the hospital, she was so angry at having been kept waiting in the emergency room for what she considered too long a time that she refused to be admitted there. Instead, she asked to be taken to the Creedmoor Psychiatric Center, in Queens Village — a state mental institution that serves the two million people who live in Queens. Miss Frumkin had spent time at Creedmoor even more recently than she had at Hillside: She had been a patient there until about two weeks earlier — from May 9, 1978, to May 31, 1978. At 4:30 A.M. on June 16, Dr. Aaronson called the psychiatric resident on duty at Creedmoor, who was handling night admissions, told him about Miss Frumkin and described her condition, and asked if it would be all right to send her to Creedmoor for an admission screening — a required procedure. The Creedmoor resident said it would, so Dr. Aaronson filled out a transfer form. At five o'clock, an emergency-room clerk called for a city ambulance, which arrived quickly. As soon as Miss Frumkin was safely in the ambulance and headed for Creedmoor, Miller drove back alone to the building where he worked. It was one of two buildings on the grounds of Creedmoor that were operated by Transitional Services for New York, Inc., a nonprofit agency that tries to help the mentally ill return to their communities. Most of the residents in the two buildings are newly discharged Creedmoor patients. The buildings had been Miss Frumkin's home from June 14, 1977, until February 5, 1978, and again from May 31, 1978, until her fall in the bathroom on June 16. Miller and Miss Frumkin returned to Creedmoor separately at five-thirty, just as the sun was rising.

Two

Creedmoor Psychiatric Center (it was officially called Creedmoor State Hospital until 1974, and is still called a mental hospital or a mental institution by many of its patients and staff) is a collection of seventy buildings scattered over three hundred acres. The first two sizable modern buildings for patients opened in 1926, and were almost immediately filled with more patients than they were certified to hold. Creedmoor remained overcrowded for the next thirty years. By 1956, the overcrowding had reached almost forty-five percent; there were 6018 patients in a hospital certified to hold 4188. There was no uniform method of treatment for Creedmoor's patients during those years. Patients in straitjackets were a common sight. Some patients were given sedatives, such as paraldehyde, a foul-smelling liquid that pacified them for a short while, or were cocooned in sedative packs — moist, cool sheets that were wrapped around the patient and then around the examining table on which he lay. The hospital's physiotherapy department treated some patients with heat lamps, massages, and whirlpool baths. The hydrotherapy department treated patients in "continuous-flow tubs," where they were immersed for hours in water. Several forms of shock treatment were introduced in the late thirties and early forties, among them electroshock therapy and insulin-coma therapy. Lobotomy surgery was introduced in 1952 — "further evidence," the institution's annual report said, "of the desire here to keep up with the modern trend in the care of patients."

In 1952, Henri Laborit, a French surgeon, observed that chlorpromazine, a newly synthesized compound of the phenothiazine family, had a remarkably soothing effect on his patients, and he suggested that it might play a role in psychiatry. Prompted by Laborit's suggestion, several psychiatrists began to use chlorpromazine on mental patients, and some small-scale testing was done in Europe over the next few months. The drug seemed successful but was still considered experimental by many authorities when the New York State Department of Mental Hygiene started to test it on a grand scale, in 1954. Mental-health professionals who had seen state-hospital wards in 1954, before Thorazine — the brand name by which chlorpromazine became known — and saw the same hospitals in 1956 found only one adjective adequate to describe the change: "revolutionary." Thousands of patients who had been assaultive became docile. Many who had spent their days screaming subsided into talking to themselves. The décor of the wards could be improved: chairs replaced wooden benches, curtains were hung on windows. Razors and matches, once properly regarded as lethal, were given to patients who now were capable of shaving themselves and lighting their own cigarettes without injuring themselves or others or burning the hospital down.

The so-called wonder drugs of psychiatry proliferated. By 1960, a number of new antipsychotic phenothiazine derivatives, with such brand names as Mellaril, Compazine, Trilafon, Stelazine, and Prolixin, had taken their places alongside Thorazine on the shelves of hospital pharmacies. By 1978, the pharmacist's armamentarium also included such antipsychotic drugs as Taractan, Navane, Haldol, and Moban, from different chemical families; such antidepressant drugs as Elavil and Sinequan; and lithium carbonate, an antimanic drug. The drugs did not cure serious mental illnesses, and not even their most ardent proponents claimed that they did. What was claimed was that the drugs controlled the florid symptoms and bizarre behavior of schizophrenia and other psychoses, much as Dilantin controlled epileptic seizures. Patients who were free of the frightening symptoms of psychotic disorders became accessible to other forms of treatment, such as psychotherapy, vocational therapy, and recreational activities. Many who had been locked up could be safely permitted to go out on the hospital grounds alone, and many whose thinking and behavior had been stabilized by the drugs — whose psychoses were in remission — could be released from the hospital.

The immediate effectiveness of the new drugs was as vividly shown by numbers as by adjectives. The New York State Department of Mental Hygiene's annual report for fiscal year 1956 stated that between April 1, 1955, and March 31, 1956, there was "a fifty-percent reduction in the amount of restraint and seclusion necessary to keep extremely disturbed patients from harming themselves or others." That same year, the number of patients in the state's mental hospitals — a figure that had been increasing by as much as 2748 a year during the previous decade — actually declined, from 93,314 to 92,862, and it kept going down every year thereafter. In 1978, there were 27,866 patients in the state's hospitals.

The drugs were most effective on first-time patients, many of whom could now be released after several months of treatment. Sylvia Frumkin, for instance, was admitted to Creedmoor for the first time in June of 1964 and was released in October of 1964. The drugs were less effective on the chronic, long-term patients — those who wound up in the hospital's "back wards." Chronic patients were in the majority then. In 1962, almost sixty-five percent of the state's mental patients had been hospitalized for five years or more, almost thirty percent for twenty years or more. Some doctors said that the psychoses of these patients didn't respond to the drugs because they were so long-standing as to be permanent. Some sociologists said that the chronic patients were at least as much the victims of the hospitals in which they had been confined as they were of the illnesses that had originally brought them to the hospitals — that they had become so "institutionalized" that they remained withdrawn, apathetic, dependent, and unable to communicate, though the new drugs may have made them calmer.

In any event, by the mid-sixties the drugs had changed the policy of New York's Department of Mental Hygiene and the policies of the mental-hygiene departments of other states. Until then, New York State had kept building more hospitals and expanding existing hospitals, such as Creedmoor, simply to keep up with the large number of people committed to its care. Once the drugs had begun to reduce overcrowding, the state's policy became one of depopulating its hospitals. After years of ignoring the journalists and sociologists who had attacked these hospitals in well-written and well-documented books, the department's every pronouncement agreed with its critics: State hospitals were hazardous to the health of mental patients. The department announced its turnabout goals of "deinstitutionalizing" the already institutionalized, of keeping the newly mentally ill from ever becoming chronic cases by deflecting admissions, and of continuing to shorten the hospital stays of those whose psychotic crises were so acute that they had to be admitted. The proper place for most mental patients, the state said, was in the community.

State and federal legislation — particularly the Community Mental Health Centers Act, passed by Congress in 1963 — called for the funding of community mental-health centers, to reduce the role of the discredited state hospitals in the care of the mentally ill, but community facilities were built slowly when they were built at all. In seeking to carry out its fresh policy in the mid-sixties, the department had to acknowledge that its large, centralized hospitals were better suited to what they had been doing in the late nineteenth century and the first half of the twentieth century — storing damaged human beings — than they were to the reverse goal of treating and releasing salvageable human beings.

Creedmoor's population decline had lagged behind the state's during the first post-Thorazine decade. Creedmoor's director, Dr. Harry A. LaBurt, believed in the old policy and in maintaining the status quo. Dr. LaBurt was an inaccessible man, who enjoyed the trappings of power. His office in Creedmoor's Administration Building was locked, and he admitted visitors by pressing a buzzer. Dr. LaBurt lived alone in the director's mansion and seemed to be more comfortable with the members of the Queens Village Rotary Club, to whom his state-provided cook tendered luncheons, than with some members of the staff. He sometimes used the word *darkies* in the presence of black Creedmoor employees.

By 1968, the atmosphere of Creedmoor's wards had improved as a result of the efficacy of the new drugs, but the institution was still essentially the pre-1955 hospital. The admissions wards, where new patients were kept, were all in one building and received the bulk of the hospital's slim professional resources. Patients who didn't improve within twelve to eighteen months in the admissions wards were sent to the back wards to share the neglect of the chronic patients. In 1966, when the median length of stay for new admissions to state psychiatric hospitals had fallen to seventy-four days, Sylvia Frumkin was admitted to Creedmoor for the second time. She stayed for twenty-seven months. After failing to respond to drugs, to electroshock therapy, and to insulin-coma therapy — which Creedmoor was the last state psychiatric hospital to stop using, and which Miss Frumkin recalls with special rage and resentment — she was transferred from the Admissions Building to a back ward. In 1968, each patient building was presided over by a psychiatrist and run on his behalf by a supervising nurse. While the ward attendants were essentially custodians and cleaners, they had the ability to make a patient's life more pleasant if they liked the patient and if the patient was well behaved and cooperative. ("Good" patients helped attendants clean up after "bad" patients and were rewarded with cigarettes or quarters or small favors for making beds, scouring floors, and washing attendants' cars.) The attendants could make life miserable for a patient they regarded as being difficult or "pesty" — an adjective that appears frequently in the records of Miss Frumkin's numerous stays at Creedmoor. Miss Frumkin remained in the back wards for several months, and spent six weeks of that time in a straitjacket. Her principal custodian was an attendant named Evelyn Deacon, a woman she has likened to Mr. Hobbs and Nurse Ratched, who are unsympathetic characters in, respectively, *I Never Promised You a Rose Garden* and *One Flew Over the Cuckoo's Nest* — two of many novels she has read and enjoyed that are set in psychiatric hospitals. Miss Frumkin's condition suddenly improved in late 1968, and she was discharged in 1969. In January of 1969, Dr. LaBurt, having exceeded the mandatory retirement age of seventy, was made to retire, despite his resistance, after more than twenty-five years of presiding over Creedmoor.

Creedmoor's new director, Dr. Irwin M. Greenberg, was a man who believed that large state hospitals such as Creedmoor should be depopulated. During the winter of 1969, the insulin unit was abolished, the admissions wards and the back wards ceased to exist, and most of Creedmoor's patients were assigned to the unit at Creedmoor corresponding to the section of Queens in which they had lived before being admitted. Each unit became a semiautonomous mini-hospital, headed by a "unit chief," or chief of service, which admitted only patients from its "catchment area." A unit had its own "treatment teams" of psychiatrists, psychologists, nurses, social workers, occupational and recreational therapists, and attendants, all of whom were supposed to know the patients in the unit; the patients were a mixture of the young and the old, the acute and the chronic. The staff was supposed to work intensively with both the regressed patients and the newly admitted, and to cooperate with the staffs of the out-patient facilities that were initially set up in the wards and then gradually relocated in the unit's geographical area to provide support for discharged patients, to keep them from being readmitted, and to keep others from ever having to become in-patients. Dr. Greenberg stayed at Creedmoor for three years. During his term, the number of in-patients decreased from 5704 to 2949, while the number of out-patients increased from none to 3000. Under Creedmoor's next director, Dr. William L. Werner, the population continued to decline; on March 31, 1978, it was 1684.

In 1978, there were some specialized units at Creedmoor for categories of patients who required specialized care. These included several large geriatrics units, for patients sixty-five and older; a small adolescent unit, for about twenty sixteen-to-twenty-year-old patients; a small forensic unit, for most of Creedmoor's thirty or so forensic patients (those who had been accused of a crime and found unfit to stand trial because of mental disease or defect, and also those who had been tried and found not guilty for the same reason); a small new unit for some of Creedmoor's multiply disabled patients (who suffered from severe retardation and psychoses, and in some cases from physical disabilities as well); and a small unit for alcoholics. The hospital's nine geographical units, however, contained about three-fifths of Creedmoor's patients. These units were called Steinway, Elmhurst, Woodside/Ridgewood, Central Queens, Clearview, Richmond Hill, Jamaica, Queens Village, and South Shore/Rockaway. The smallest geographical unit had an average of seventy in-patients in 1978, and the largest an average of a hundred and fifty. The population of Queens is predominantly white, and Creedmoor's in-patients reflected its demographics.

In 1972, New York State upgraded the job descriptions and civil-service standing of the attendants in its mental hospitals and gave them new titles: mental-hygiene assistant therapy aides, or M.H.A.T.A.s, and mental-hygiene therapy aides, or M.H.T.A.s. At Creedmoor, the staff and the patients turned both abbreviations into the word *mahatas*. To Miss Frumkin, who was between her third and fourth stays at Creedmoor when the titles were changed and the word was coined, *mahata* conjured up a combination of Indian elephant keepers and Brahman sages. The M.H.A.T.A.s and M.H.T.A.s are now called mahatas, attendants, and therapy aides interchangeably. Whenever Miss Frumkin and many other white patients are angry, however, they call them "nigger bitches." By 1978, the great majority of attendants at Creedmoor were black women. Irish, Italian, and German men and women had predominated in the wards in the 1930s and 1940s, but most of them had retired. The number of white women applying for these low-paying jobs had dwindled by the 1950s. (In 1978, an assistant therapy aide's starting salary was $7800 a year. A therapy aide's starting salary was $8700 a year.) There was a dearth of male applicants of any race. Men who could score well on the civil-service test for therapy aides could usually score well on the civil-service tests for city policemen or sanitation men, or for safety officers on Creedmoor's security force; all of these were better-paying positions.

The color line of economic and educational disparity in America showed up again when one reached the upper strata of the hospital's staff. In 1978, the social workers, psychologists, occupational and recreational therapists, treatment-team leaders, and unit chiefs were predominantly white, American-born, and American-educated. The psychiatrists, on the other hand, were mainly foreign-born and foreign-educated. For decades, it had been impossible to attract many American-born and American-educated psychiatrists to Creedmoor. In the 1940s, a number of European psychiatrists who had fled Hitler had gone to work in state hospitals after immigrating to the United States. A number of these psychiatrists had stayed on, but in the late 1970s most had reached or were about to reach retirement age, and were being replaced primarily by Asians, who preferred the stability and economic promise of life in America to the risks of practice in their underdeveloped and often turbulent homelands. Language and cultural frame of reference have thus been problems in psychiatrist-patient relationships at Creedmoor since the 1940s. Some of the Europeans had learned to speak and write English well. Others had not. With the increase in Asian psychiatrists, the difficulties were revived — often in a more severe form, because of the greater cultural differences. On May 9, 1978, when Miss Frumkin began her most recent previous stay at Creedmoor, she had been admitted by Dr. Felix Koppel, a native of Czechoslovakia, who spoke and wrote English fluently. On May 31, 1978, when Miss Frumkin was ready to go from Creedmoor to Transitional Services, she had been discharged by one of his colleagues, Dr. Sun Ming Wong, a Chinese. Dr. Sun frequently used masculine pronouns in referring to his female patients. The day he discharged Miss Frumkin, he told her parents, "The patient he is doing good."

⸙ ⸙ ⸙

Between eight o'clock in the morning and four-thirty in the afternoon, the hours when almost all the members of the professional staff were on duty at Creedmoor in 1978, each geographical unit screened its own prospective patients for admission. From four-thirty in the afternoon to eight in the morning, when the geographical units didn't have registered nurses on duty, much less psychiatrists, admission screenings were done on the second floor of Building 40, an ugly seventeen-story high rise that serves as the hospital's medical building, and it was there that Miss Frumkin was taken just before 6:00 A.M. on June 16, 1978.

She was seen immediately by a nurse and by Dr. Anand Khanna, the psychiatric resident on night duty. (In June of 1978, Creedmoor had twenty-two psychiatric residents, most of them foreign-born.) Dr. Khanna read the papers that had accompanied Miss Frumkin from L.I.J.-Hillside, observed her, and asked her a number of questions. Like Dr. Aaronson, Dr. Khanna found Miss Frumkin oriented in respect to time, place, and person; subject to swings in mood; and suffering from severely limited insight and judgment. She admitted to him that she heard God's voice, and made a few statements ("Everyone's out to get somebody somehow") that he characterized as paranoid delusions. His impression of her condition was "schizophrenia, paranoid type." Although Miss Frumkin denied having any suicidal or homicidal ideas, Dr. Khanna decided that she required hospitalization, because he judged her to be "dangerous to self."

In 1978, there were two primary criteria for admission to a state psychiatric hospital in New York: being considered dangerous to others — homicidal or assaultive — and being considered dangerous to oneself. The dangerous-to-self category included the suicidal and also people like Miss Frumkin, who had now been found by two psychiatrists to be too incapacitated to survive in the community. In earlier decades, people who expressed such common psychotic symptoms as delusions (firm, fixed ideas maintained against logical argument and despite objective contradictory evidence) or auditory or visual hallucinations (false sensory perceptions in the absence of actual external stimuli) were readily admitted to Creedmoor and were sometimes kept there for years; but by 1978 it was state policy for harmless psychotics to be treated in their communities.

Dr. Khanna asked Miss Frumkin if she wanted to sign a voluntary-request-for-hospitalization form. She said that she did. The form has a seven-line space in which a person who is applying for voluntary admission to Creedmoor is instructed to state his or her reasons for requesting hospitalization. Miss Frumkin wrote three short words in a chicken-scratchy handwriting: "I need rest." (If she had been brought to Creedmoor, had refused to sign the form, and had been found in need of immediate hospitalization, she could have been hospitalized involuntarily, as she had been on more than one occasion in the past.) Dr. Khanna asked Miss Frumkin what medication she had been taking. She told him she had been taking two hundred milligrams of Moban daily — a moderately high dose of one of the newer antipsychotic drugs. Dr. Khanna prescribed the same medication for her but suggested on the doctor's order sheet he filled in that the medication be revaluated by the doctor in the ward to which Miss Frumkin was to be sent for screening several hours later.

The nurse in Building 40 gave Miss Frumkin a brief physical examination. Her temperature, pulse, and blood pressure were normal; her height was five feet four inches and her weight was 152 pounds. The nurse also saw to it that the blood and urine tests and the chest X ray ordered by Dr. Khanna (a routine part of Creedmoor's admissions procedure) were completed. Miss Frumkin was handed a cardboard folder about Creedmoor called "Information About Your Hospital," which she stuffed into her bag, and a form that explained her status and rights as a voluntary patient, which she signed without reading because she already knew her rights by heart. Miss Frumkin knew that at any time after admission, a voluntary patient could request his or her release, in writing, from the director of the hospital. Within three days, the director's surrogates either had to release the patient or, if they believed the patient to be in need of further hospitalization, had to seek a court order to retain the patient against his or her will. In practice, letters from voluntary patients requesting release within seventy-two hours went to their psychiatrists, who were most familiar with their cases. If a psychiatrist believed that a patient needed additional, involuntary treatment in the hospital, he would ask a colleague to examine the patient. If the colleague agreed with his appraisal of the patient's need for continued hospital care, the patient would be kept at Creedmoor while an application for a court order of retention was made. The New York State Supreme Court for Queens County held sessions at Creedmoor — in Building 40 — once a week. Every voluntary patient had a right to a court hearing and a right to be represented at the hearing, free of charge, by a lawyer provided by the Mental Health Information Service — a court agency, independent of the Department of Mental Hygiene, which had been set up in 1965 to help safeguard the constitutional rights of patients.

Miss Frumkin had given Transitional Services as her address. Transitional Services was in the catchment area of the Queens Village unit. At eight o'clock, when the day shift reported for duty at Creedmoor, she was taken to the patient building in which the Queens Village unit was situated. She spent a short time there. The Clearview unit's catchment area, in northeastern Queens, includes Flushing, Bayside, and Beechhurst, where Miss Frumkin's parents live, and she had been a patient in the Clearview unit from May 9 to May 31. According to hospital procedures, most patients who returned to Creedmoor within ninety days of release were sent back to the unit from which they had been discharged, to be screened for readmission.

Not long after Clearview's unit chief, Hermine Plotnick, came to work, at eight o'clock on June 16, she received a call from a member of the staff of the Queens Village unit. Mrs. Plotnick was told that Queens Village had Miss Frumkin and would be bringing her over shortly. When Miss Frumkin was discharged from Clearview to Transitional Services on May 31, Mrs. Plotnick had been afraid that she wouldn't be able to cope with the strain of living in that less restrictive setting. Mrs. Plotnick knew that Miss Frumkin had a long history of "decompensating" — deteriorating to a psychotic condition — under what she thought to be pressure, but Mrs. Plotnick was disappointed that she had been able to stay off the ward for only two weeks.

A great deal of Mrs. Plotnick's time in 1978 was spent on administrative duties. In addition to being responsible for Clearview's in-patient unit — which in 1978 was the hospital's second most populous geographical unit, with an average of 146 patients a day in its four locked wards — she was also responsible for the Clearview Motivation Center, the Clearview Day Center, and the Clearview Out-Patient Clinic. Mrs. Plotnick is a small, dark-haired woman in her early fifties. When she took the test for unit chief, in 1973, her score was the fifteenth-highest in the state, and when she took the test for deputy director, in 1976, her score was the highest in the state. She is a prompt, efficient administrator; she usually puts in a ten- or twelve-hour workday after getting up at five-thirty in the morning to play one of two grand pianos in her living room. She is intolerant of those in her unit who don't work a full eight hours. As a consequence of her busy schedule, she didn't come to know all of Clearview's in-patients, but she did come to know most of the long-termers and the multiple recidivists such as Miss Frumkin.

Miss Frumkin had been one of the first patients whose name was brought to Mrs. Plotnick's attention just before she became Clearview's unit chief, on February 28, 1974. On February 27, Mrs Plotnick had met with her predecessor to discuss the immediate problems she would be inheriting. One of her first duties was to handle a case involving Miss Frumkin and a therapy aide who had slapped her in January of 1974 and had been brought up on charges of patient abuse. (The aide was ultimately disciplined.) Miss Frumkin had been released from Creedmoor in April of 1974, before Mrs. Plotnick, who was caught up in the details of taking over and reorganizing her new unit, had a chance to meet her; but Miss Frumkin had returned to Creedmoor, and to the Clearview unit, in February of 1976, and had remained there until her first discharge to Transitional Services, in June of 1977.

During that sixteen-month period, Mrs. Plotnick had become well acquainted with Miss Frumkin. Miss Frumkin was the sort of person who stood out in a crowd — even a crowd of patients on a psychiatric ward. Mrs. Plotnick and numerous members of her staff found her both more exasperating and more pathetic than most of the other Clearview patients. She was so exasperating because the acute phases of her psychotic episodes (during which she often struck staff members and provoked them to the point of rage, though less often to the point of striking back) lasted much longer than those of most patients, and because even when she was not in an acute phase she was arrogant, nasty, and demanding. She seemed pathetic because the difference between what she was and what she might have been was so much greater than it was for most patients. Sylvia Frumkin's older sister, Joyce, was a well-known and well-paid executive with one of New York's most elegant department stores, and Joyce's success rankled her younger sister. Mrs. Plotnick suspected that Sylvia Frumkin could have had a glamorous career if she hadn't spent so much of her life as a mental patient. Sylvia's flamboyance reminded Mrs. Plotnick of Auntie Mame; her verbal facility and stridency brought Bella Abzug to mind. Even as a patient, Miss Frumkin sought the limelight and often found it. In 1977, she was one of only a dozen patients whom Dr. Werner saw individually once a week for hourly psychotherapy sessions. He had heard about Miss Frumkin and had thought that he could help her, even after so many other doctors had failed.

Although Miss Frumkin was first diagnosed as a schizophrenic and considered ill enough to be hospitalized when she was fifteen, in 1964, almost a decade after Thorazine and some of the other new drugs had worked their wonders on thousands of chronic schizophrenics and newly diagnosed schizophrenics, the drugs had worked only limited wonders on her. By 1977, numerous doctors at numerous hospitals had prescribed numerous doses of numerous medicines and combinations of medicine for her. "My blood is nothing but chemicals," she had cried out on a hundred occasions. The antipsychotics, the antidepressants, and the antimanic drugs had helped her over her acute episodes and had stabilized her, but they had never brought her to the point where she could function independently in the community; she had never been able to hold a full-time job, for example, and she couldn't stay out of a psychiatric hospital for long, even without the pressure of having to earn a living. Miss Frumkin was one of an unfortunate minority — an estimated fifteen percent of all seriously ill mental patients — who are "treatment-resistant." It had distressed Dr. Werner as well as Mrs. Plotnick, both of whom knew Miss Frumkin's case history, to see how much her condition had deteriorated by 1977. After her first Creedmoor hospitalization, which lasted four months, she had been able to finish high school. After her third hospital stay, in 1972, she had been able to finish medical-secretarial school. Since then, the course of Miss Frumkin's life had been all downhill. Her periods of acute psychosis lasted longer; she functioned at a lower level during each remission; the intervals between her hospital stays were getting shorter. Even when she was in Creedmoor — during the sixteen-month period from early 1976 to mid-1977, for example — her mental state went up and down like a seesaw. So did her weight. Sometimes she weighed 125 pounds, sometimes 175.

Miss Frumkin's weight was the first thing Mrs. Plotnick noticed when she saw the Queens Village therapy aide with Miss Frumkin in tow in the secretaries' office of the Clearview unit, at 9:45 A.M. on June 16, 1978. Miss Frumkin had been overweight when she was discharged two weeks earlier — several other patients had called her Hippopotamus — and now her hips seemed to bulge out even more than they had then. The zipper of her skirt couldn't stand the strain; it was halfway open.

When Miss Frumkin saw Hermine Plotnick, she embraced her. She blurted out a rapid-fire account of her fall and talked quickly and angrily about how she had been kept waiting at Hillside. She was logged into Clearview's screening book. Mrs. Plotnick said that she would take Miss Frumkin to the screening. The Queens Village therapy aide left after giving a secretary the papers she had brought with her. Mrs. Plotnick took the papers with her free hand. She was holding her key ring in the other: Creedmoor employees and their keys are rarely parted, and most employees jangle as they walk. She used the largest of seventeen keys — a passkey that fits almost every ward door in the hospital — to open five locked doors that she and Miss Frumkin encountered on their way to a room called the chart room, where all admission screenings for the Clearview unit were conducted.

It was ten-thirty by the time a psychiatrist, a nurse, and a social worker — the team that was to screen Miss Frumkin — were seated around a long table in the center of the room. Miss Frumkin was already seated at the table, fidgeting in a plastic chair, crossing and uncrossing her legs, talking to herself, and occasionally laughing, as if in response to something that had been said to her by someone nobody else in the room could see. She took no notice of two other people in the room at the time: a second psychiatrist, who was joking with a patient, and a therapy aide, who was talking on the telephone to a patient's husband.

In 1978, two psychiatrists alternated admission screenings in the Clearview unit — Dr. Shamaldaree Batra (the man who was joking with the patient) and Dr. Sun Ming Wong, the psychiatrist who had discharged Miss Frumkin on May 31 as a "he." It was Dr. Sun's turn to do an admission screening. While Miss Frumkin fidgeted and addressed invisible presences, Dr. Sun skimmed the papers that Mrs. Plotnick had handed him: ten or twelve pages about Miss Frumkin's experiences in the L.I.J.-Hillside emergency room, her transfer to Creedmoor, Dr. Khanna's admission note, and her reception in the Queens Village unit. Dr. Sun was a thirty-five-year-old native of Taiwan who had received his medical degree in Taipei, had come to the United States in 1973, had begun his residency in New Jersey, and had completed it at Manhattan Psychiatric Center, the state hospital that serves Manhattan. He had come to work at Creedmoor, and at Clearview, during the summer of 1977, when Miss Frumkin was at Transitional Services for the first time. He was not familiar with her case. He had discharged her in May only because the psychiatrist who had been routinely seeing her was then caring for patients in another ward. While Dr. Sun was skimming Dr. Aaronson's consultation form, Miss Frumkin was still talking out loud to no one in particular. "I'm not a nut," she said. "I have something wrong with my brain. The attendants here are good, but sometimes they're overworked, and they take it out on the patients. At Hillside hospital, we had something to do all day. We had a patients' newspaper, the *Rehab Rap*. Money has its place." Miss Frumkin got up, sat down again, recrossed her legs, rummaged through her handbag, looked at an electric clock on the wall, hummed a few bars of a song from *Annie,* and rambled on. "Everybody needs sex," she said. "I haven't had sex for five years. The clock is in this room because they want patients to learn how to tell time. I know Mary Poppins, and she lives in Massachusetts. I didn't like the movie *Mary Poppins*. They messed up the book so they could try to win the Oscar. Movies come from real life. This morning, when I was at Hillside, I was making a movie. I was surrounded by movie stars. The X-ray technician was Peter Lawford. The security guard was Don Knotts. That Indian doctor in Building 40 was Lou Costello. I'm Mary Poppins. Is this room painted blue to get me upset? My grandmother died four weeks after my eighteenth birthday." Miss Frumkin laughed.

When Miss Frumkin stopped talking and laughing, Dr. Sun tried to ask her a few questions about her fall and some questions similar to the ones she had already been asked by Dr. Aaronson and Dr. Khanna: her name, the date, the place.

After telling him, irritably, that her name was Sylvia Frumkin, that her friends sometimes called her Sylvie, that her enemies sometimes called her Silly, that as a child her enemies had called her Pumpkin Frumkin, that it was June 16, and that she was in Creedmoor State Hospital, she declined to answer some of his other questions. Instead of saying yes, she had recently thought of committing suicide, or no, she had not, she delved into her bag, pulled out the cardboard folder about Creedmoor she had been given in Building 40, and began to read aloud from it, interjecting her own comments between sentences.

" 'Philosophy of Treatment,' " she read. " 'The individual with a problem is best served in his own environment.' I'm against polluting the environment, always have been. 'This is the basic philosophy of the New York State Department of Mental Hygiene and of Creedmoor Psy. Center.' They shouldn't use abbreviations. Abbreviations can drive mental patients nuts because they don't know what they mean. 'If he leaves his home to be hospitalized, it is harder for him to return to his former life.' Amen. 'However, for the few who do need hospitalization, these facilities are available and every attempt will be made to allow the client privacy, dignity, and comfort.' Privacy? Dignity? Comfort? Bull. All untrue. They're killing people here."

When Miss Frumkin stopped reading, Dr. Sun made another attempt to interview her. She wasn't the least bit interested in talking about her fall and its aftermath. "To hell with your questions; I'll say what I want to say," she said, raising her voice. After releasing a stream of profanity, she shouted a series of rhetorical questions at Dr. Sun, the nurse, the social worker, and Mrs. Plotnick: "Do you know what it's like to keep coming back here? What torture it is to be sent through the revolving door again and again? The pain, the suffering, do you know how it hurts?" Hermine Plotnick reflected that since January of 1978 Miss Frumkin had gone from Transitional Services to Hillside, then to Creedmoor, then to Transitional Services, and then back to Creedmoor — that the door had already revolved four or five times for her in 1978 and the year had more than six months to go. Mrs. Plotnick softly told Miss Frumkin that she understood, and that she sympathized with her suffering. The more softly she spoke, the more furious Miss Frumkin became. "Why are you talking so softly?" she shrieked. "I can't hear you! Let me talk!" And talk she did, insulting Mrs. Plotnick, Dr. Sun, the nurse, and the social worker with another explosion of invective. The social worker tried to soothe Miss Frumkin, with results similar to Mrs. Plotnick's. "I've never had a T-shirt, and I've always wanted one, damn it," Miss Frumkin cried. "A pink one or a white one. Size medium. Dwight Miller works for the KGB. So does my father." Miss Frumkin stopped shrieking and started to mumble.

Mrs. Plotnick noticed that Dr. Sun was already filling out the papers necessary to admit Miss Frumkin to Clearview. A small percentage of the people who are admitted to Creedmoor during the night are "screened out" when they are rescreened during the day. Someone who may have been upset enough to hit his next-door neighbor in the evening may have calmed down after spending the night in Building 40. A unit social worker can telephone day-treatment centers, day hospitals, and out-patient clinics that aren't open at night, and, after also getting in touch with relatives, can arrange for the person to live at home with the support of one or another of the resources in the community. Miss Frumkin, however, given her condition then, was not a nighttime admission who could be diverted during the daytime. In the mental-status report that Dr. Sun wrote on her, he first briefly recapitulated the events of June 16. He then wrote, "Pt. appears to be very agitated and restless so formal interview seems to be not obtainable at present time. Her verbal production is markedly increased with flight of ideas ["flight of ideas" is defined in a standard psychiatric glossary as "verbal skipping from one idea to another; the ideas appear to be continuous but are fragmentary and determined by chance"] as well as marked loosening of association. Her motor activity is also increased. Mood is labile. Affect is inappropriate. [In psychiatry, "affect" and "emotion" are commonly used interchangeably. An "inappropriate" affect is one that is obviously discordant with the content of the individual's speech — for example, laughing after mentioning the death of one's grandmother.] Thought content is highly fragment and illogic. Sensorium unimpaired. [Miss Frumkin was obviously aware of her surroundings. In psychiatry, simple words are never used where complicated ones will do.] No delusion or hallucination could be elicited, also suicidal and homicidal ideation is not examined." Dr. Sun diagnosed Miss Frumkin as a manic-depressive, manic type. Though disturbances of both thought and mood are characteristics of schizophrenia and manic-depressive illness, schizophrenia is defined as a psychosis in which disordered thought is the more prominent symptom, and manic-depressive illness is defined as a psychosis in which a disordered mood is the more prominent symptom.

More than one person in the chart room at the time of Miss Frumkin's screening who later happened to read Dr. Sun's mental-status report was surprised that he believed he had failed to elicit any delusions or auditory hallucinations from Miss Frumkin, but, as Dr. Sun later acknowledged, he didn't recognize the names Mary Poppins, Don Knotts, Peter Lawford, and Lou Costello, and he hadn't understood that Miss Frumkin had said anything about making movies with these people, whoever they were. Those who read the report were even more surprised by Dr. Sun's diagnosis, and later asked him about it. He said he had based his diagnosis on three of the main symptoms he had observed: increased motor activity; pressure of speech (rapid, accelerated, frenzied speech that sometimes exceeds the ability of the vocal muscles to articulate and at other times exceeds the ability of the listener to comprehend); and flight of ideas. These three psychotic symptoms are listed in definitive textbooks on psychiatry, and in the third, and latest, edition of the American Psychiatric Association's *Diagnostic and Statistical Manual of Mental Disorders* (*DSM-III*), as three of the primary symptoms of a manic episode. Two of the other psychotic symptoms that Dr. Sun had observed and recorded — inappropriate affect and loosening of associations — are listed in textbooks on psychiatry as among the main symptoms of schizophrenia.

It is not unusual in the field of psychiatry for three psychiatrists to see a person within a period of seven hours — as Dr. Aaronson, Dr. Khanna, and Dr. Sun had seen Miss Frumkin — and to offer three different impressions or diagnoses based on interviews lasting an hour or less. If the practice of medicine is an art in which science is employed, then the field of psychiatry may be the branch of medicine with the most art and thus the greatest room for disagreement. There are no definitive tests for schizophrenia, as there are for pregnancy or syphilis. Psychiatric diagnoses are based on interpretations of symptoms, and the symptoms are not always symptomatic of the same underlying cause. It may be impossible to distinguish between an acute psychosis brought on by amphetamine abuse and an acute schizophrenic psychosis: the patient's symptoms often appear identical. What may strike one psychiatrist as "loosening of associations" may strike another as "flight of ideas." In addition, cultural biases can result in conflicting diagnoses. From 1967 to 1970, Dr. Barry Gurland and Dr. Joseph Zubin, both of the New York State Psychiatric Institute, in Manhattan, supervised a study to determine why such a large percentage of mental patients in the United States were diagnosed as schizophrenics, while in Great Britain statistics showed a higher percentage to have manic-depressive disorders. The question was whether the variation in the occurrence of these psychoses in the two countries was due to ethnic or social factors, or was simply one of diagnosis. The study made use of videotapes of American patients in American hospitals and English patients in English hospitals, to enable doctors in the two countries to diagnose the illnesses of the same patients. After three years, the conclusion was that the difference was one of diagnosis. European psychiatrists claim that their American counterparts diagnose schizophrenia too often, and accuse the Americans of being afflicted with "schizophrenomania."

Doubt has been cast on all psychiatric diagnoses by periodic and well-publicized instances of sane journalists who have feigned psychoses in order to gain admittance to mental hospitals to do "inside" stories about their stays. Some of the journalists, having once been admitted, and having collected sufficient material for their exposés, had a difficult time establishing their sanity when they wanted to get out to write about the miseries they had experienced. Further doubt has been cast on psychiatric diagnoses by the frequency of disagreement in forensic cases. In New York State, as elsewhere, those accused of murder and other crimes can avoid prison sentences if they successfully plead not guilty "by reason of mental disease or defect"— insanity, that is — at the time the act was committed. The defense is normally one of last resort, and it is used in only about two percent of the criminal cases decided by juries, because the consensus among trial lawyers is that jurors are reluctant to believe it. "The phrase 'not guilty' sticks in their craw," an eminent courtroom performer, F. Lee Bailey, once explained. The insanity defense is thus attempted mainly in homicide cases where there is convincing proof that the accused did the killing. When it is employed, however, the defense attorney never seems to have difficulty producing a forensic psychiatrist to testify that the alleged murderer was mentally ill at the moment of the act, regardless of how sane he may appear to be in the courtroom; and the prosecutor, with equal ease, finds a forensic psychiatrist who says that the defendant was and always had been sane. When the insanity defense succeeds, it usually provokes controversy.

In 1978, Creedmoor's most widely known patient was a thirty-three-year-old New York City policeman in its forensic unit named Robert Torsney. Just before midnight on Thanksgiving of 1976, Torsney and another officer in a patrol car were sent to investigate a report of an armed man at the Cypress Hills housing project in the East New York section of Brooklyn. They did not find the man. As the two policemen were leaving the building, six black youths approached them. One of the young men stopped to ask Torsney a question. Torsney drew his .38-caliber service revolver, shot the youth point-blank in the head, reholstered the pistol, and continued walking back to the patrol car. He subsequently admitted that he did not like blacks. Randolph Evans, fifteen years old, died after several hours in a hospital. Torsney testified at his trial for second-degree murder a year later that he had drawn his weapon and fired because he had seen the young man pull from his waistband a shiny object that appeared to be a gun. His fellow-officer and other witnesses testified that they had seen nothing resembling a gun, and none was ever found. The defense that Torsney's attorney adopted was that, as he put it to the jury, "if there was no gun, this man is sick." The attorney found a psychiatrist — Dr. Daniel Schwartz, director of forensic psychiatry at Kings County Hospital Center, in Brooklyn — who testified that Torsney suffered from a rare form of organic mental illness called psychomotor epilepsy, and that at the moment he shot Evans he had been in the midst of a "psychomotor seizure." The psychiatrist who testified for the prosecution — Dr. Herbert Spiegel, a professor of clinical psychiatry at the Columbia University College of Physicians and Surgeons — said that Torsney appeared to have a neurotic character disorder that gave him a tendency to panic in situations where he imagined he was being threatened, and that this emotional flaw could have led him into "a mistaken perception" that Evans was pulling a gun. Dr. Spiegel said, however, that he could find no evidence of psychomotor epilepsy or any other indication that Torsney was psychotic, as distinguished from neurotic. Torsney was legally sane, the prosecution's psychiatrist said, and was thus responsible for his actions. Until Torsney killed Randolph Evans, he had never been known to fire his revolver on duty, and he had an unblemished record of eight years on the police force. The jury, all whites, chose to believe Dr. Schwartz, not Dr. Spiegel. They acquitted Torsney "by reason of mental disease or defect."

In December of 1977, right after the trial, Torsney was sent to Mid-Hudson, in New Hampton, New York, one of several maximum-security psychiatric facilities that the state maintains for forensic patients and for particularly violent patients transferred from other psychiatric hospitals, such as Creedmoor. The psychiatrists at Mid-Hudson who examined Torsney were unable to find the rare epileptic condition on which the defense psychiatrist had based his diagnosis and the jury its verdict. They could not discover any other psychosis, either, and, in March of 1978, having decided that Torsney was not dangerous, they had him transferred for further examination to the forensic unit of the hospital serving his home community. Because Torsney lived in Queens, that hospital was Creedmoor. The law in New York State says that a person acquitted by reason of mental disease or defect must be committed to a mental hospital until it can be determined that he or she is no longer a danger to self or others — a determination that can be made in as little as sixty days. The individual can then be released if a judge accepts the determination of the psychiatrists at a court hearing.

The psychiatrists at Creedmoor, like those at Mid-Hudson, could not find any indication that Torsney was psychotic. In July of 1978, the chief of Creedmoor's forensic unit initiated proceedings to release him. That December, after a nine-day hearing, a judge ordered Torsney released. The order was immediately stayed by a higher court at the request of the Brooklyn Attorney's office, and was reversed on appeal by the higher court in February of 1979. The judges ordered Creedmoor to devise an "individual treatment plan" to help Torsney "surmount his dangerous personality disorder." The Department of Mental Hygiene, in turn, appealed the case to the state's highest court, the Court of Appeals, arguing, in effect, that the judges were unwilling to face up to a miscarriage of justice within their own system, and were attempting to turn the mental hospitals into penitentiaries in a misguided effort to rectify it. "If he's not clinically ill," William Carnahan, the attorney who was in charge of the appeal for the Department of Mental Hygiene, asked, "what are you going to treat?" In July of 1979, the Court of Appeals set Torsney free, in an angrily divided four-to-three decision.

Torsney had by then been a patient for about a year and a half in Mid-Hudson and Creedmoor. Creedmoor had been allowing him to go home to his wife and children most nights and weekends since December of 1978, and had continued the policy despite the changing rulings from the courts. A spokesman for the hospital said that the treatment team responsible for Torsney had recommended letting him spend most nights and weekends with his family as part of a rehabilitative program. The chief of Creedmoor's forensic unit said that the courts could not legally accuse the hospital of releasing Torsney unless he was permitted to stay out beyond forty-eight hours. A report by the Department of Mental Hygiene in February of 1978 showed that the median hospital stay of one-quarter of the murder defendants in the state acquitted by reason of mental disease or defect between September 1, 1971, and June 30, 1976, had been less than a year. Torsney had in the meantime been seeking to retire from the Police Department with a $14,000-a-year medical-disability pension, on the ground that a psychiatrist and a jury had declared him subject to a mental disease or defect, and thus unfit for duty. However, a departmental trial — a police disciplinary proceeding — had found no evidence of the rare form of epilepsy on which the acquittal was based. Torsney's request for retirement and a $14,000 pension was rebuffed, and he was dismissed from the force in June of 1979, on the charge that he had "without provocation shot and killed" Randolph Evans. Jack Ruby, the killer of Lee Harvey Oswald, had also sought to gain acquittal by claiming that he had shot Oswald during a psychomotor-epilepsy seizure. His jury had not believed the defense experts.

One purpose of *DSM-III* is to dispel diagnostic controversy and confusion by more precisely defining schizophrenia, manic-depressive disorders, and most other mental disorders. The manual seeks to spell out with greater specificity the criteria for making a diagnosis, because a diagnosis can have certain treatment implications. The standard textbooks in psychiatry stress the importance of knowing a patient's history in order to make a correct diagnosis. On June 16, 1978, Dr. Sun did not have Sylvia Frumkin's written case history; the records of all her previous admissions to Creedmoor and summaries of her stays in other mental hospitals were in Clearview's central files and had not been retrieved in time for the screening. If Dr. Sun had read Miss Frumkin's history, he would perhaps have decided, as Dr. Werner and almost all the other psychiatrists who had treated Miss Frumkin over the years had done, that hers was a textbook case of schizophrenia. She had first been hospitalized at the age of fifteen. For most schizophrenics, the age of onset for the disorder is adolescence; for manic-depressives, it is usually early adulthood or later. Schizophrenics tend to progress to a state of mental deterioration, the downhill course that Dr. Werner had observed in 1977; manic-depressives remit between psychotic episodes, often appear normal to strangers, are able to hold good jobs, and do not progress to a state of mental deterioration. Even when Miss Frumkin was at her best, as she was during part of her first stay at Transitional Services, in 1977, strangers saw that there was something peculiar about her and wouldn't hire her even for menial jobs; she had applied for jobs as a waitress in 1977 and had been turned down.

Conflicting diagnoses were less important before lithium carbonate became available for psychiatric treatment in the United States. Lithium, a simple metal ion that was first used in the treatment of mania in Australia, in 1948, is the oldest of the modern antipsychotic drugs. It was not commercially produced in the United States until 1970. Before 1970, the same antipsychotic drugs had been used to treat both schizophrenia and mania. Lithium carbonate made differential diagnoses critical, because it is the drug of choice for the treatment of mania, and is also used preventively in the treatment of recurrent mania and depression; it is effective about eighty percent of the time. On June 16, 1978, it turned out not to matter for the moment that Dr. Sun had diagnosed Miss Frumkin as a manic-depressive, because he had no intention of giving her lithium then. What he was most concerned with on that day was her extreme agitation and excitement. On the page of the doctor's order sheet that had been begun by Dr. Khanna, Dr. Sun prescribed Thorazine injections to control Miss Frumkin's agitation. She was to be given a 50-milligram injection immediately and 50-milligram injections every four hours "PRN" (as necessary) to counter the agitation. Thorazine, the first of the wonder drugs, is still one of the two or three antipsychotics with the greatest sedative effect, and is regarded by some authorities on psychopharmacology as the drug of choice not only for acute schizophrenia but for acute mania as well, because it takes effect more rapidly than lithium does. Dr. Sun did not reevaluate and change Dr. Khanna's order prescribing for Miss Frumkin 200 milligrams of Moban in 50-milligram oral doses four times a day. Dr. Sun was taking the afternoon off, and he had some other patients to attend to before leaving the ward for the weekend.

Once Dr. Sun had screened Miss Frumkin for Clearview,

Hermine Plotnick left the chart room and returned to her office, and the social worker and the nurse went back to the work they had been doing before Miss Frumkin's screening. A therapy aide made up a chart for Miss Frumkin. The aide put the papers from Hillside, from Building 40, and from the Queens Village unit into a metal chart holder along with the Khanna-Sun doctor's order sheet. She also put in several blank forms for future use: some "Progress Note" forms, which would be filled out mainly by the therapy aides on the three shifts who would be observing Miss Frumkin, and some "Treatment and Medication Record" forms, which nurses and medication-certified therapy aides were required to initial each time they administered medication to Miss Frumkin. In the months ahead, other pieces of paper would thicken Miss Frumkin's chart: a page to record her weight; an account by Transitional Services' Dwight Miller of her fall in the bathroom; the results of periodic lab tests. Once Miss Frumkin's chart had been hung on a rack in the chart room, the therapy aide escorted her to the state-clothing room.

Many people admitted to the Clearview unit kept the clothes they were wearing when they came in, and also all the possessions they had brought with them. If newly admitted patients were wearing nice clothes, as Miss Frumkin was on the morning of June 16, 1978, and if it appeared that they would be unlikely to take care of their clothes and to protect their other belongings from theft, the therapy aides locked up their clothes and their belongings in the ward's private-clothing room. The therapy aides then let new patients choose clothes from the state-clothing room to wear in the ward until their condition improved. The clothes in the state-clothing room included not only underwear and other garments that the state bought in quantity and distributed to the wards but also clothes left behind by previously discharged patients. Some of the latter were outfits that the discharged patients had acquired at the Creedmoor Boutique, a shop on the hospital grounds where patients were periodically entitled to replenish their wardrobes, free of charge. The Boutique offered a combination of newly purchased state garments and donations. On June 16, Miss Frumkin chose a green T-shirt and a pair of green polyester pants, size 16, from the state-clothing room. She recalled having worn this outfit during her stay at Clearview in May. The pink skirt and blouse she had worn upon admission (which a therapy aide had specially selected for her in the Boutique to wear the day she was last discharged), her poncho, her octagonal-framed eyeglasses, and her mother's Timex watch were locked up for safekeeping. Miss Frumkin kept her pocketbook. After she had changed her clothes, she walked with the therapy aide to the women's dayhall, where she sat down in an easy chair. The therapy aide left, and Miss Frumkin soon started carrying on an animated conversation; she was talking either to herself or to her phantom voices.

Paulette Finestone, a homely young woman who had met Miss Frumkin at Creedmoor many years before and who had occasionally gone out for lunch with her when they were both out of the hospital at the same time, approached Miss Frumkin. She listened to her for a couple of minutes. When there was a lull in Miss Frumkin's chatter and laughter, Miss Finestone greeted her old acquaintance.

"Hi, Sylvia," she said. "Welcome home."

"Get lost," Miss Frumkin replied.

Three

On June 16, 1978, the Clearview unit, which was to be Miss Frumkin's home for most of the remaining months of the year, occupied the first floor of a three-story building of custard-colored brick known as N/4. (The Jamaica unit was on the two upper floors.) Building N/4 was opened in 1932. It is a grimy building that appears at first glance not to have aged well, a building of which one might say that it had seen better days — unless one chanced upon a photograph of N/4 taken the year it opened. One would then have to say that it was a building that had had no better days. Although N/4's grubby exterior is enhanced by a few turrets and Corinthian columns, the building's predominant architectural features are its drab bricks, its squat mass, and its enormous barred and screened windows and barred porches, which make the playful Moorish and Greek touches easy to overlook. Some people who have passed N/4 daily for years are so distracted by the screams, cries, and laughs coming from the building that they have never noticed its architectural amenities.

N/4 is shaped like two U's that are connected at their bases by short hallways to a slightly longer I-shaped central corridor. In 1978, each U contained two of Clearview's four wards. Wards 041 and 042 were in one U, and wards 043 and 044 were in the other. Opening off both sides of the central corridor were the offices of some of the Clearview personnel whose work had to do with the whole unit. The offices were Spartan, with state-issue metal desks, and had such graphic bureaucratic reminders as a "5 74" stenciled in black on the light-blue wall leading into the secretaries' office to show when it was last exposed to the brushes and rollers of the painters on the state payroll. Sometimes the employees tried to decorate the offices with plants they brought from home — to no avail, for the plants were quickly stolen. So, periodically, was the electric clock on the wall of the secretaries' office.

A short distance past these offices, to the left and the right, two locked metal doors led to the wards; the door on the right led to wards 041 and 042, the door on the left to 043 and 044. If one walked past these metal doors and continued down the central corridor, one passed other rooms — a dental clinic, a conference room, the office of Nutrition Services, the office of Clearview's medical nurse — and eventually reached N/4's ambulance entrance. In June of 1978, Creedmoor had two ambulances, which were summoned when patients were injured, fell sick, or (on rare occasions) died, and had to be taken to Building 40 or to the Queens Hospital Center, one of two city hospitals in Queens. Creedmoor's patients are sent to the Queens Hospital Center or to other medical facilities for any physical problems that the staff in Building 40 cannot handle — from abortions that patients want to surgery and treatment for such serious diseases as cancer and kidney trouble. The ambulances at Creedmoor are not celebrated for the speed with which they respond to calls — especially calls received around the change of shift. At four o'clock on the afternoon of October 13, 1978, a pugnacious Clearview patient named Alexander Morton was attacked by another Clearview patient. Morton collapsed on the floor of the 044 dayhall. A therapy aide who was close by telephoned for an ambulance at 4:02. While waiting for the ambulance to arrive, Dr. Sun and other members of the staff gave Morton, who was unconscious and was bleeding from the mouth, mouth-to-mouth resuscitation. When his vital signs continued to deteriorate, Dr. Sun also gave him an injection of epinephrine, a heart stimulant. The ambulance arrived at 4:30. Dr. Sun, a Clearview nurse, and an oxygen tank accompanied Morton on the ambulance ride to Building 40, where he was pronounced dead on arrival. He had probably died on the floor of the ward.

Wards 041 (male) and 042 (female) housed chronic patients, and were euphemistically known as the rehabilitation side, and wards 043 (female) and 044 (male) housed new patients and readmitted patients, and were known as the admissions side. Each side had about a dozen mentally retarded and multiply disabled patients. These patients didn't belong on either side of Clearview, or, for that matter, at Creedmoor, but in June of 1978 there were few alternative facilities for them. Some of these patients were quiet, and, because they created no problems, they were the patients most often ignored at Clearview. Others, who were disruptive, could not be ignored, and they caused a good deal of mischief and sometimes real grief. One patient in 044 was a skinny, intractable, profoundly retarded, assaultive young man named Kevin Kiernan. He had a misshapen head, little usable language, and a penchant for biting. He refused to wear anything but pajama bottoms except on the one day every month or two that his mother visited him, when he permitted her to dress him. He usually lay on the dayhall floor holding a magazine. He occasionally became violent — especially when some new and acutely psychotic patient tried to touch his magazine. He had persistently bitten the ear of a psychotic male patient several years earlier. The ear had healed badly.

Albert Rosenthal, another profoundly retarded Clearview patient with only a few words in his vocabulary, was perhaps the saddest example of Creedmoor's inability to care for unfortunates of his kind. For his own protection, Rosenthal had to be kept in a glass-free environment. Whenever he saw glass, he broke it and injured himself. Once, when he was in a dining room at Creedmoor, he had cut himself with a glass salt shaker. Since 1974, he had lived in a seven-by-nine-foot room near the Clearview chart room. His cell-like quarters contained a bed and a commode. He spent most of the day sitting on his bed or on the floor rocking back and forth silently. When he was upset, he banged for hours on the room's locked door. Creedmoor's psychiatrists were periodically instructed to gradually terminate the medication of all patients who had been hospitalized for five years or longer; it had been found that a number of them improved when their medication was lowered or stopped. Some got worse, however. In 1978, after Rosenthal's medication was lowered, he pulled out all his fingernails and toenails. On June 16, 1978, while Dr. Sun was screening Miss Frumkin, Rosenthal's mother was in her son's room with her other child, Gail — also a Clearview patient. Gail, who hardly spoke, either, had been diagnosed as autistic and profoundly retarded as a child (properly diagnosing patients who don't talk is even more difficult than diagnosing those who do), but since she didn't break glass she spent her days in the ward, rocking back and forth in a chair. Mrs. Rosenthal took her children out on the Creedmoor grounds on Wednesday afternoons. She came to the hospital every Friday morning to take them home for the weekend and returned them to Creedmoor on Monday morning. When her children were at home, they were kept in the Rosenthals' glass-free basement; Mrs. Rosenthal and her husband would often take turns staying awake with them. Members of the staff called Tuesdays and Thursdays Mrs. Rosenthal's "days off." She often told Mrs. Plotnick that she worried about what would happen to her children after her death. Mrs. Plotnick worried about what would happen to Mrs. Rosenthal if Albert and Gail predeceased her. Members of the staff had often advised Mrs. Rosenthal to spend more time on her own life. "You don't seem to understand," she had replied. "This is my life."

The women's dayhall to which Miss Frumkin had been taken by the therapy aide — the dayhall of Ward 043 — was a vast, high-ceilinged room, sixty-eight feet long and twenty-three feet wide. It had nine large, barred windows and a floor of linoleum tile in a gray-and-black checkerboard pattern. The fluorescent lights on the ceiling often flickered; they seemed to expose the dreariness of the dayhall rather than to brighten the room. The white paint on the ceiling was peeling. The walls, which had been painted a cheerful shade of yellow, were soiled.

In 1976, one of Creedmoor's volunteer workers had decorated a section of the long inner wall with a mural meant to depict a fairy tale. According to the artist, the central figure in this fairy-tale landscape, a woman dressed in a red-and-gold gown and a medieval-style pointed headdress, was a princess. According to a number of the patients in 043 who suffered from religious obsessions, the central figure was the Virgin Mary. The mural also depicted a white unicorn with a garland draped around its neck, and a multicolored snake wrapped around a tropical tree. The artist had hoped that the mural would soothe the patients. It often had the opposite effect. On June 16, 1978, one of the most disturbed people in 043 was a young woman named Barbara Herbert. Like Kiernan, Mrs. Herbert had a penchant for biting. She had left her teeth marks on quite a few patients during each of the many occasions she had been at Creedmoor. Mrs. Herbert was a short, attractive Jewish woman in her early thirties with peroxide-blond hair; she had a daughter, who had been placed in foster care, and a husband, who often threatened to divorce her before, during, and after her stays in the Clearview unit. She paced the floor in front of the mural on June 16 and shook her fist at the princess, whom she addressed as Mary. "Jesus is *my* child," she shrieked to the princess figure, pounding her fists on the red-and-gold gown. Pointing to the princess and shifting her angry gaze to the snake, she addressed it. "Tell *her* to get out of the Garden of Eden!" she yelled.

Except for the mural, the walls of the dayhall were almost bare. There was nothing else on them but a small wooden board that read "This is Creedmoor Psychiatric Center"; two notices about the Mental Health Information Service; a clock; two No Smoking signs (the injunction was never enforced); and two fans. The fans were in motion on summer days whenever their cords had been repaired by Creedmoor's small maintenance department after the latest troubled patient had cut them. On June 16, one fan swirled the hot, stale, smoky air. The only air conditioner in the Clearview unit was in Mrs. Plotnick's office.

Set into one of the dayhall's short walls was a TV, protected by a locked Plexiglas shield. The television set was on a good deal of the time, except when Kiernan or another agitated patient had sneaked in behind a therapy aide who had unlocked the plastic shield in order to tune the set, switch channels, or turn the set off or on, and pulled the knobs off, leaving the patients with no television for the week or two it took for the set to be repaired. The dayhall was furnished with a water fountain, an area rug, two plastic plants, two cigarette urns, several hassocks and wastebaskets, a few coffee tables, three or four small tables, and four Formica room dividers, which were too small to divide the great rectangle of the dayhall and stood in it looking lost. There were also a dozen chairs, half a dozen love seats, and several sofas — an assortment of plastic-and-metal and upholstered pieces in different shapes and colors that had little in common except multiple cigarette burns. There were rarely enough chairs and sofas to go around. The cleaner assigned to 043 and 044, a friendly woman who was pleasant to the patients and was well liked by them, mopped the dayhall floor conscientiously every weekday. She labored in vain. The floor became sticky with spilled soda and coffee, and powdery with cigarette ashes, ten minutes after the latest wet mopping. The ward smelled of coffee, stale cigarette smoke, and unwashed and incontinent patients.

A door along the dayhall's outer wall led to a barred porch. The door was almost always kept open during the daytime, when the weather was good. On the porch were another dozen mismatched and worn plastic chairs and a long table. Patients who spent time on the porch, and those who sat on the porches of the Jamaica unit above, tossed cigarette butts, soda cans, bottles, clothes, paper, and other trash out through the widely spaced bars. The littered grass within throwing range of the porches resembled a vacant lot in a slum neighborhood. When patients on the porch looked south, past the unsightly refuse and pieces of broken glass, and across Creedmoor's once well-tended and now uncut lawns, and through the dying branches of its untrimmed trees, they could see and hear the cars and buses of the outside world going up and down Hillside Avenue, about seventy-five yards away. On hot summer days, the patients could hear not only the traffic but another sound — the cries of seagulls scavenging for food on the scruffy lawns; and they might feel a breeze drifting in from Long Island Sound, a few miles away as the seagulls flew.

Partway down the long inner dayhall wall, where the therapy aides on duty usually sat at a small table, was an archway. Under the archway to the left was a large bathroom, which served the women patients in 043. It was outfitted with eight washbasins (with dripping faucets), six toilets, two showers (for which the shower curtains came and went like the clock and the plants in the secretaries' office), and several mirrors. The bathroom looked and smelled like a big restroom in a busy turnpike restaurant on the third day of a four-day holiday weekend: no better, no worse. Toilet paper and soap were often scarce, and there was a shortage of towels and sanitary napkins. Over the years, Miss Frumkin had grown accustomed to drying herself with a sheet after taking a shower at Creedmoor. Mrs. Plotnick observed on her daily inspection rounds in June of 1978 that although three of the six toilets had doors and three had curtains, all had seats. Some years earlier, Creedmoor's toilets often lacked seats. It was assumed that the employees were stealing them, simply because most of the patients seemed to lack the skills to fence them. In 1978, a stereo set vanished from Clearview, and a five-gallon beverage dispenser disappeared the first day it was used.

Employee theft, a recurring problem at Creedmoor, became public knowledge rather dramatically a few years ago when a Creedmoor attendant and her small child were held at gunpoint by the attendant's common-law husband in their apartment. When the husband got tired, the attendant tied several sheets together, attached them to a radiator, threw the sheets out the window, climbed out with her child, and slid safely to the ground. The police had been called, and several television crews were at the scene. The following day, her escape showed up on the evening news telecast. The words *Creedmoor State Hospital* were easy to read where they had been stamped on her makeshift rope hanging from the window. One November, some years earlier, half the turkeys that were to be cooked for the patients' Thanksgiving dinner were stolen; replacement turkeys had to be procured and cooked in haste.

In June of 1978, Creedmoor's Safety Department, which was in principle responsible for investigating such thievery, consisted of one chief, three sergeants, and twenty-four safety officers. Their duties also included patrolling the grounds to look for patients who had escaped from their units; helping attendants subdue violent patients; checking the locks on the doors of the various buildings in which food and other valuable commodities were stored; and keeping the peace in two dormitory-like buildings in which some seventy employees lived in small rooms with communal bathrooms. The Safety Department kept a daily log of its routine patrols and of unusual happenings. Its 1978 log showed that there had been no falloff in employee theft to match the decline in patient population. On January 31, a kitchen was broken into and 285 pounds of chicken, 105 pounds of ground beef, 40 pounds of turkey, and 30 pounds of coffee and sugar were taken. On February 5, another kitchen lost six cases of cooked beef, 60 pounds of diced beef, 45 pounds of ground beef, and a slicing machine. The following month, that same kitchen lost 115 pounds of sliced ham. Five days after that, 100 pounds of ham, 120 pounds of frankfurters, and 24 pounds of turkey and veal vanished from a third kitchen. One safety officer, who refers to the Safety Department as "the Keystone Cops," was asked if any of the meat was recovered. "No burglary at Creedmoor has ever been solved," he said.

A corridor led from the women's dayhall to the women's dormitory. Off this corridor were the offices of some of the staff assigned to the 043-044 side of Clearview — a social worker's office, a psychologist's office, and the ward office, which was the office of the person in charge of a shift. One of the rooms off this corridor — a room that measured seven feet by nine — had a metal door with a small plastic viewing panel; on the floor was a mattress, and there was a large window at the back, protected by a metal grille inside and by bars outside. This was the "seclusion room," in which a disturbed patient could be kept. On occasion, a patient put in the seclusion room was so distraught that he banged his head against the wall and hurt himself. There were four seclusion rooms in the Clearview unit, one for each ward. Mrs. Plotnick had repeatedly requested protective padding for one of them. (Some of Creedmoor's other units did have padded seclusion rooms by 1978.) Her requests for padding went unheeded, and she resented the bureaucratic indifference to her patients. At Creedmoor in 1978, there were no more

Evelyn Deacons with the power to lock a Sylvia Frumkin up or put her in a straitjacket for six weeks. (Straitjackets were rarely used at Creedmoor in 1978.) Only a doctor could order a patient into seclusion, and for a period no longer than two hours; the doctor could renew the order every two hours if he felt that continued seclusion was necessary. When a patient was ordered into seclusion, the door to the room was locked. If a patient felt upset and asked to go into the room, its door was left unlocked, and the room was referred to as a quiet room or an isolation room.

The women's dormitory, at the end of the corridor, was a rectangular space about the same size as the dayhall. The dormitory was divided by archways into four many-windowed sections, called cubicles. Each cubicle contained from three to eight beds and several wardrobes. There were almost always enough beds to go around; when there were not, patients slept on the floor. The door to the dormitory was kept open at night, so that patients could use the nearby night toilet, but it was usually kept locked during the day. Almost all of Creedmoor's patients were on psychotropic drugs, and the medication made many of them drowsy — particularly for the first few days. Given a choice, they would have spent a good part of the day in bed. They were not given a choice. The patients were made to get up at six o'clock in the morning, unless a doctor granted an exemption, so that the night shift could help them make their beds and get them dressed and ready for breakfast before going off duty. They were not permitted to go to bed before eight o'clock in the evening, except, again, on those infrequent occasions when a doctor prescribed daytime bed rest for a patient. If the patients were permitted to sleep during the day, they would be up a good part of the night. Some of them — those who slept during the day on the furniture and floors in the dayhall, the porch, and the corridors, and those who were extremely agitated — were up anyway. The patients who were up at night disturbed not only the majority of the patients, who wanted to sleep, but also the midnight-to-eight-thirty shift, some of whom liked to sleep on duty.

A seventy-foot corridor separated the women's dayhall from the men's dayhall. Opening off to the left of the corridor was a spacious dining room. The two dayhall doors at either end of the corridor were usually kept open during the daytime, so that the men in 044 could mingle freely with the women in 043. Coed dayhalls had come in with "unitization," in 1969. Dr. Greenberg, Creedmoor's director then, maintained that patients came from a heterosexual world and would be returning to one, and that the dayhalls should approximate conditions on the outside as closely as possible. Almost every heterosexual act that took place in the outside world in 1978 took place in the dayhalls, porches, bathrooms, dormitories, offices, and corridors of the Clearview unit in 1978; so, for that matter, did almost every homosexual act.

The men's dayhall was similar in dimensions and furnishings to the women's dayhall. Another corridor connected the men's dayhall with the men's dormitory, and it too was lined with offices — among them the offices of Dr. Sun and Dr. Batra, the chart room in which Sylvia Frumkin had been screened, a treatment room (where medication was stocked, poured, and dispensed when it wasn't dispensed in the dayhalls near the water fountains), and two seven-by-nine-foot unpadded rooms. One of these rooms was permanently occupied by Albert Rosenthal; the other was used as a seclusion room. The men's dormitory in 044 closely resembled the women's dormitory in 043. The bars over the windows in both dormitories went halfway up; the top halves of the windows were covered only with screens. The men showed a greater proclivity than the women for climbing up and tearing the screens, and periodically did so. Before dawn on June 3, 1978, a male patient escaped through a window in the men's dormitory. The window's torn screen was reported to the maintenance department that day. It wasn't fixed on June 4. Another patient escaped through the torn window screen on the evening of June 5. On June 6, the maintenance department was again informed of the situation, but the window wasn't repaired on that day, either, supposedly because of a shortage of maintenance workers.

Wards 041 and 042, where chronic patients were kept, were similar to wards 043 and 044, even down to the periodically broken window screens, through which some of the men in 041 also made their exit during 1978.

⁂

On June 16, 1978, the day Miss Frumkin was readmitted, the admissions side of the Clearview unit was theoretically allocated thirty-four employees, who were supposed to be taking care of twenty-three acutely ill women and thirty-five acutely ill men. Besides Miss Frumkin, Kevin Kiernan, Albert and Gail Rosenthal, Barbara Herbert, and Paulette Finestone (who had been brought to the ward one day in late March from Clearview's out-patient clinic, which she had been attending, after biting one of three relatives who had accompanied her to the clinic, hitting the clinic nurse on the head, and turning over a table on the clinic psychiatrist's foot), the other patients in wards 043 and 044 also had grave troubles. There was Hiroku Izutsu, a beautiful young Japanese woman who had once burned down the children's psychiatric ward of one of Manhattan's best-known voluntary hospitals. Miss Izutsu had been transferred from that burned-out ward to Creedmoor's adolescent unit, had graduated to Clearview, and, on June 16, 1978, went around asking questions like "Is the ridiculous still normal?" There was Isabelle Holzman, an attractive young single woman who was eight months pregnant and almost catatonic. (She had her baby in July and returned to Clearview in an agitated psychotic state in October.) There was Deirdre Gerrity, an extremely obese woman of fifty-nine (she was five feet seven and weighed 220 pounds), who had been admitted to Creedmoor in late April. Miss Gerrity was a retired nurse who had never been in a psychiatric hospital before; her sister had reluctantly brought her to Creedmoor because she could no longer care for her at home. Her psychiatric diagnosis was psychosis with arteriosclerosis. Her medical examination upon admission showed that she was suffering from high blood pressure, varicose veins, edema in both feet, severe degenerative arthritis of the entire lumbar spine, anemia, severe dermatitis, and heart trouble. With all these physical ailments, it was painful for Miss Gerrity to move. She didn't want to eat. It took two or three therapy aides to lift her out of bed or out of a chair, so that she could be helped to the toilet, to the shower, or to the dining room. Sometimes eight hours went by on the day shift without anyone moving her. The evening shift often complained about the condition in which the day shift had left Miss Gerrity. The night shift complained that she was nasty and refused to help herself and said that she wanted to go to a private hospital, where she felt she belonged. Miss Gerrity gave the employees on all three shifts the impression that she had lost her will to live. Her physical condition continued to deteriorate. In late July, she was transferred to Building 40; in early October, she died of congestive heart failure.

There was a middle-aged retarded man named Richard Moscow, who at least twenty times a day conducted the same dialogue with the Clearview therapy aides and with patients and visitors who knew his life story:

Moscow: When's my daddy coming?
Aide: Your daddy died a few years ago.
Moscow: When's my mommy coming?
Aide: Richard, you know your mommy died a few years ago, the same week as your daddy.
Moscow: When's my brother coming?
Aide: Soon, I hope, Richard, soon.

There was a man whose parents had left New York and moved to another state, leaving no forwarding address. About two-thirds of the patients on the chronic side and many of the retarded patients on the admissions side never received any visitors and never stopped feeling their absence. The patients in 043 and 044 were young and middle-aged, alert and confused, well-educated and illiterate. Their only common denominator was the fact that they shared a statistical misfortune: Each year, more than a million and a half people in the United States become patients in psychiatric facilities.

If on paper thirty-four employees seemed inadequate to attend to the needs of the fifty-eight patients in wards 043 and 044 through the twenty-four hours of June 16, the paper ratio looked a great deal better than the real one in the wards. There were twenty people assigned to the day shift (eleven therapy aides, nine others), seven to the evening shift (six therapy aides and one licensed practical nurse), and seven to the night shift (all therapy aides). Five of the day shift's professionals — two psychiatrists (until Dr. Sun left for the day, at noon), one treatment-team leader, one nurse, and one social worker — were on the payroll and on the premises on June 16. One typist was also present. The three other professionals allocated to the unit — a licensed practical nurse, a psychologist, and a rehabilitation specialist — were not there, because they existed only on paper. The three people who had held these jobs had left earlier in the spring, and replacements had not yet been hired.

Of the eleven therapy aides assigned to the day shift, only four were on the premises on June 16, one of whom had arrived an hour and a half late. Three therapy aides were taking their regularly scheduled days off; two were on vacation; one was out on a personal-leave day; and one therapy aide had been suspended on May 30 on disciplinary charges of abusing a patient. (She remained out for almost two months, until the case was settled.)

From nine-thirty in the morning to four in the afternoon, the four therapy aides had to cover the 043 and 044 dayhalls and porches. This meant that, at best, one aide was trying to cover the 043 dayhall and porch and a second the 044 dayhall and porch. The two others were off on coffee breaks or lunch breaks or were engaged in other tasks. The four took turns going back and forth to Building 40 to escort patients to scheduled appointments at the X-ray department, the dermatology clinic, or the ophthalmology clinic. They also had to go to Building 40 to take specimens to the laboratory or to pick up medication at the pharmacy. Even when all four therapy aides were in the N/4 building, some were in the chart room writing progress notes on the patients' charts, in the treatment room giving medication, or in the ward office answering the telephone, rather than in the dayhall.

On June 16, 1978, the consequences of understaffing were a greater-than-usual neglect of patients and a greater-than-usual harassment of staff. On February 1, 1979, understaffing had a somber result. Of seven therapy aides who were scheduled to work the evening shift (from 4:00 P.M. to 12:30 A.M.), five called in sick. The evening-shift supervisor asked a young woman on the day shift to work overtime. While the three therapy aides were getting the patients to and from the dining room, handling a regularly scheduled telephone hour for the two wards, between six and seven o'clock, and preparing the evening medication, a young man named Lloyd Colvin went out to the 043 porch. The door to the porch was open. Colvin had come to Creedmoor on January 31, with his mother. When Dr. Sun screened Colvin for admission, he had asked him if he had a history of suicide attempts or of drug or alcohol abuse. Both Colvin and his mother had denied that he had ever tried to commit suicide or that he was a "substance abuser." Dr. Sun had almost not admitted Colvin — he had thought that the young man might be able to continue living at home and be treated in an out-patient facility — but the mother had prevailed upon him to admit her son for a short stay. When Colvin went out to the porch on the evening of February 1, he got up on a chair, took off the heavy work boots he was wearing, tied the boots' sturdy laces together, looped the laces around his neck, attached the loop to the porch bars, stepped off the chair, and hanged himself. He had last been seen by a therapy aide in the dining room at five-forty, and by the evening supervisor around six-fifteen. He was dead by the time two patients went out to the porch and found him hanging there, at five past seven, and summoned the only therapy aide in the dayhall, the young woman working overtime. This therapy aide and the evening supervisor cut Colvin down. Hermine Plotnick believes that people who are determined to commit suicide will sooner or later succeed in doing so. She also believes, however, that if there had been adequate staffing of the evening shift on 043 and 044 on February 1, 1979, Colvin might have been discovered sooner and might have survived. The day after Colvin's death, his chart came over from the hospital's central files. It revealed that he had a history of suicide attempts and of drug and alcohol abuse. Mrs. Plotnick says that if these facts had been known, he might have been more carefully watched at Clearview. After Colvin's death, the doors to Clearview's porches were locked at dusk.

Four

It was after eleven o'clock in the morning on Friday, June 16, by the time Miss Frumkin had been screened for admission by Dr. Sun, had changed into state clothes, and had taken a chair in the women's dayhall. After shooing Paulette Finestone away, she remained seated for a while, seemingly oblivious of everything and everyone around her. But not for long. Soon she was on her feet, hurrying over to the nurse on duty. She demanded to use the telephone. When the nurse told her she would have to wait until another patient had finished making a call, Miss Frumkin screamed at her. The nurse escorted her to the telephone a few minutes later. Miss Frumkin dialed the extension of Dr. Werner, Creedmoor's director. She tried to tell Dr. Werner's secretary her troubles, but became incoherent. The nurse and a therapy aide had to struggle with her to get her to put the telephone down. The nurse, who had been at the admission screening, then led Miss Frumkin to the treatment room and tried to give her the injection of Thorazine that Dr. Sun had ordered that she be given immediately for agitation. Miss Frumkin refused the injection. She said she would take Thorazine orally instead. The nurse poured Thorazine into a paper cup and handed it to Miss Frumkin, breaking a rule that requires written permission from a doctor to substitute one form of a drug for another. Rules were broken hundreds of times a week in the Clearview unit. This knowledge didn't sit easily with Mrs. Plotnick, who is a perfectionist, but there was little she could do except to rail periodically against the difference between the way things were at Creedmoor and the way she thought they ought to be. Between sips of the bad-tasting Thorazine, Miss Frumkin called the nurse a jerk, a slut, and a dodo. After Miss Frumkin's insults became threats and she started to hit the nurse, the nurse went to Dr. Sun, caught him just as he was leaving, and got him to write out a seclusion order, which went into effect at twelve-fifteen. Once Miss Frumkin had been put in the seclusion room, she flopped down on the mattress as if she were relieved to be there. A few minutes later, a therapy aide brought her lunch on a tray. Miss Frumkin, who had been mumbling unintelligibly, took the tray, wolfed down the food, and handed the tray back. She soon lay down and dozed off. When the seclusion order expired, at two-fifteen, the door to the room was opened. Miss Frumkin was asleep. She was left in the room to sleep, with the door open.

Miss Frumkin awakened shortly before four, but she appeared content to stay in the quiet room. Around five o'clock, she felt hungry, got up, and walked into the dayhall. When the door to the dining-room corridor was opened, she went into the corridor and stood in line with the other patients, whispering to herself. Dinner at Clearview was usually served at five-twenty. Like breakfast and lunch, the meal was served cafeteria-style. Each patient took a tray, a plate, and eating utensils, and walked past a counter. Food-service workers positioned behind the counter doled out portions of some foods; patients helped themselves to others.

The dining room that served the patients on Clearview's admissions side was a bright, buff-colored room with tables for four. There were containers filled with plastic flowers on the tables. The dining room was a moderately attractive place when it was empty. It was not an attractive place at mealtimes. Many of the patients — Miss Frumkin was one of them — ate sloppily and in great haste. A few patients were so dejected that they ate little or nothing. Therapy aides helped those who could not feed themselves. Sometimes there were forks, knives, and spoons in the dining room; sometimes (after a patient had used forks and knives as weapons) there were just spoons. The food was what one might expect at a state institution with a computerized food plan (pot roast was on the menu fifty-two times a year, not fifty-one or fifty-three times) and a food budget of a dollar and sixty-seven cents per patient per day. Vegetables that were considered "expensive and exotic"— asparagus, cauliflower, Brussels sprouts, broccoli — were never served. "Extended" (casserole-type) dishes were served often: They were inexpensive and filling. The menu was nutritious, starchy, easy to gain weight on, and inflexible. Diabetic patients could get tea and coffee without sugar, but no patient could get coffee without milk, no matter how much he or she desired black coffee. Half an hour was allotted for each meal. Most patients spent ten minutes in the dining room. Some years earlier, an attempt had been made to slow the meals down — to prolong them from half an hour to an hour — so that patients could relax and chat more. The attempt had been a failure. Instead of chatting more when they were made to sit together longer, they had fought more. Clearview's patients appeared glad to eat and run, and the dining-room employees, many of whom were grouchy, appeared glad to have them do so — especially at dinnertime, so that they could go home early.

After shoveling into her mouth three helpings of everything served at dinner on June 16, Miss Frumkin returned to the dayhall, settled into an easy chair, and watched television quietly. At nine o'clock, she took the fifty milligrams of Moban that Dr. Khanna had prescribed for her. A therapy aide on the evening shift let her watch TV until ten-thirty before taking her into the dormitory, where the other women were already asleep. She assigned Miss Frumkin an empty bed next to a window. Clearview's beds had foam-rubber mattresses. Two-thirds of the mattress rested on unspringy lattice springs; the remaining third rested on two storage drawers built into the foot of the bed. Neither these drawers nor the wardrobes in each cubicle had locks; many patients slept clutching their pocketbooks. The pillows were covered with a water-repellent material rather than with soft ticking, and were unpleasantly hard. Although Miss Frumkin had had little sleep in the last thirty-six hours, she wasn't tired. She got into bed without taking her clothes off and lay quietly under the sheets and under the bedspread, which the therapy aide had forgotten to remove.

A few minutes after the night shift came on duty, Miss Frumkin got out of bed. She walked hurriedly down the long corridor from the dormitory to the dayhall. She then headed back toward the dormitory, but stopped at the employees' lunchroom when she saw a short, stocky black woman named Bernice Parrott sitting there. Mrs. Parrott was one of the 12:00-to-8:30 therapy aides assigned to 043 and 044. Miss Frumkin told her that there was some water on the floor of the dayhall and asked her if she had a mop. When Mrs. Parrott replied that she didn't, Miss Frumkin warned her that if she didn't mop up the water she would report her to the night supervisor. Mrs. Parrott asked Miss Frumkin to go back to bed, and said she would take care of the water. Mrs. Parrott went into the dayhall, found a puddle of urine on the floor, and went to the utility room to get a mop. When she returned to the dayhall carrying the mop, she found Miss Frumkin standing a few feet from the puddle. Miss Frumkin ordered Mrs. Parrott, at the top of her voice, to clean up the dayhall. Before Mrs. Parrott could clean anything, Miss Frumkin ran over to her and demanded the mop. Mrs. Parrott held on to the mop with all her strength, fearful of what Miss Frumkin would do with it if she got her hands on it. Miss Frumkin grabbed Mrs. Parrott's dress, struck her several times on the head with her fist, kicked her, and tried to bite her, screaming "Nigger, I'll nix you!" as she fought to gain possession of the mop. Mrs. Parrott was in pain, but she whirled around, pinned Miss Frumkin against a wall, pried herself loose, and ran to the nearest telephone, which was in the ward office. She hurled the mop through an open door to the employees' toilet, in the far corner of the office, picked up the telephone, and called the night supervisor, who was in the secretaries' office in the central corridor watching some members of the night shift sign in. Meanwhile, with her free hand Mrs. Parrott continued to fend off Miss Frumkin, who had followed her into the office and was still after the mop. Mrs. Parrott and Miss Frumkin wrestled; Mrs. Parrott succeeded in bringing Miss Frumkin to the floor and was able to hold her until the night supervisor came to her assistance.

Because there were no registered nurses on duty at Clearview or in Creedmoor's other geographical units during the evening and night shifts, one or two nurses, members of Creedmoor's "nurse management team," responded to calls for help from the units between four o'clock in the afternoon and eight in the morning. When the night supervisor saw Mrs. Parrott and Miss Frumkin engaged in combat, she telephoned the nurse management team. While the night supervisor was on the telephone, Miss Frumkin managed to struggle to her feet. She tried unsuccessfully to snatch the telephone away from the night supervisor. By the time the registered nurse arrived, within a few minutes of being called, Mrs. Parrott and the night supervisor had put Miss Frumkin into an empty seclusion room. Miss Frumkin was banging furiously on the door of the seclusion room. The nurse telephoned the doctor on night duty (the resident who handled night admissions was the only doctor on call for all the geographical units at Creedmoor from four-thirty in the afternoon to eight in the morning), and he gave her a verbal order to put Miss Frumkin in seclusion for two hours. Mrs.

Parrott and the night supervisor helped the nurse hold Miss Frumkin down so that the nurse could give her the Thorazine injection for agitation, as Dr. Sun had ordered. The nurse was supposed to take Miss Frumkin's vital signs before giving her the injection — if a patient's blood pressure is low, an injection can cause hypotensive shock — but Miss Frumkin was so agitated that the nurse couldn't take her vital signs. Miss Frumkin remained agitated all night. The doctor renewed her seclusion order three times. When the day shift reported to work, she was still agitated, and so received another injection of Thorazine.

⸙ ⸙ ⸙

Miss Frumkin was let out of seclusion at eight-forty-five, after receiving her Thorazine injection. She spent most of Saturday, June 17, in the dayhall, sometimes snoozing, sometimes screaming at the therapy aides and the patients. She took the Moban tablets she was given without protesting. They didn't seem to have any effect on her. She became upset again on Saturday evening. She took her clothes off, refused to go to bed, banged on many of the doors in the ward, kept the other patients awake, and insisted that she needed a blood test, because she might be pregnant. At eleven o'clock, she was given an injection of Thorazine and was put into seclusion. The nurse management team was called over twice to help with her; the doctor on night duty renewed the seclusion order twice. Miss Frumkin spent the night singing, laughing, and talking to herself.

On Sunday morning, Miss Frumkin was again let out into the dayhall. She was quiet for a few hours and then became disruptive. She took her clothes off in the men's dayhall. Irving Frumkin came to visit but soon left, because his daughter refused to pay any attention to him. She required injections of Thorazine at five o'clock and at eleven-fifteen, and spent another noisy night in seclusion, banging on the locked door.

After Miss Frumkin was let out of seclusion on Monday

morning, June 19, she ate a substantial breakfast, swallowed her morning Moban tablets complacently, and bounded into the dayhall. She was wearing the green T-shirt and green pants she had been wearing since Friday morning, but no shoes and no bra. The soles of her feet were black. Within a few minutes of entering the dayhall, she had borrowed four hair curlers and a tube of bright-red lipstick from two other patients. She spent a long time rolling a few strands of the hair in the center of her head around each of the four curlers. She applied the lipstick to her face until every inch of it was covered except her eyes. Some of the patients stared at her and laughed; others stared and gave no sign of having seen anything out of the ordinary. Then Miss Frumkin talked for an hour, nonstop, to some of the other patients, to some of their visitors, to the therapy aides, to the cleaner, to laundry workers and dining-room employees and other people who passed through the ward, and to herself. One of her soliloquies, delivered at Indianapolis 500 speed, was peppered with the names of actors, television stars, pop and rock singers, and past and present historical and political figures, as well as with brand names. It began like this: "Hitler did a good job. He cleaned up the streets. He invented the Volkswagen. I love Darth Vader. I am Darth Vader. I figured out that Mayor Koch is Charles Nelson Reilly. Adolf Hitler is forgiven. He invented methadone and the Mercedes-Benz. It was all a price war. I'm Tania and I have the biggest house in the country. Bess Myerson was originally the Statue of Liberty. I married Neil Diamond a long time ago." She grabbed the shirts of two male patients standing near her. "Elvis Presley, this is John Travolta. I've been married to Geraldo Rivera for fifteen years. The ultimate doll is Roald Dahl. Dahl. Dahl. Dahl." Sometimes Miss Frumkin got stuck on a word or a cluster of words, like a needle on a scratched phonograph record. "As I was saying, as I was saying, Dahl, Dahl, Dahl," she repeated until she slipped into the next groove. This time, she retrieved the word *ultimate.* It got her going again in third gear. "I have the ultimate question: Are we going to bring back the Edsel?" She walked over to the TV, where a few people were watching a quiz show. "Ultimate television set, is that the Thanksgiving Parade?" She stood in front of a woman who was watching TV, blocking her view of the quiz show. "Are you wearing Ultima makeup by Revlon? The man who gave me this beautiful haircut is Jason. He's the ultimate hairdresser, trust me. Dahl was the ultimate television host." Miss Frumkin walked over to a therapy aide. "How do you like my new hairstyle?" she asked.

The therapy aide shook her head in dismay as she looked at the four hair curlers and the red-lipstick war paint. "Why'd you put that stuff on your face, honey?" she asked.

"Because I wanted to look like you," Miss Frumkin answered.

The therapy aide went off and returned with some cold cream and some absorbent cotton. She stood next to Miss Frumkin and wiped a little bit of lipstick off one cheek. "I went to high school with you, but I didn't know it at the time," Miss Frumkin said, backing out of face-cleaning range with considerable agility. She recited a poem:

> Mary had a little watch.
> She swallowed it, it's gone.
> Now everywhere that Mary goes
> Time marches on.

Vainly pursuing her with the cotton and the cream, the therapy aide said, "Sylvia, did you make that up?"

Miss Frumkin's expression became quizzical. "I don't know if I made it up or if I read it in a greeting card," she said, and she scurried off, her pretty gray eyes still surrounded by an expanse of lipstick.

For the next five minutes, Miss Frumkin was a perpetual-motion machine, marching, pacing, jogging, and trotting all over the ward. She ran down the long corridor from the women's dayhall to the men's dayhall and then ran back. She occasionally stopped to ask a patient if she looked like him or her today. Most of the patients — Travolta and Presley among them — ignored her or walked away as she approached them. Sometimes a patient shouted "Stop staring at me," or "Don't look at me like that!" at her. One patient told Miss Frumkin that she was the greatest show on earth. A visitor said to the patient she was visiting, "You may be sick, but you're not sick enough to be locked up with people like that. Get yourself together so you can get out of this snake pit." Miss Frumkin grabbed one patient's hand and said, "I'm scared." The patient's hand went limp until she let go of it. She kissed a male patient on the mouth and elicited no response. She took her T-shirt off, revealing ponderous breasts. She called the therapy aide who eventually came over to put her T-shirt back on "Miss Priss." She sprinted out to the porch, where a patient was writing in a diary and two visitors were chatting with another patient. She grabbed the diarist's fountain pen, getting an ink blotch on one of the visitors' dresses in the process. She didn't apologize to the woman for staining her dress; she didn't seem to have even noticed the ink stain. She asked the other visitor for a pencil, accepted it without thanks, and tossed the pen and the pencil out through the bars of the porch. "There," she said, with satisfaction. "I've planted a pen-and-pencil tree." She went back into the dayhall, bummed a cigarette from a patient who appeared afraid not to let her have it, lit it with a lighted cigarette she had pulled out of another patient's mouth, put the cigarette back in the other patient's mouth, and started to smoke. "The moon is made of cigarettes," she said. "A tobacco leaf just jumped out of my hair." She took five puffs on the cigarette and threw it on the dayhall floor. Two other patients swooped down to pick it up and started to fight over it. Miss Frumkin walked across the dayhall, threw her arms around a rabbi, who was visiting a patient, and begged a half-empty paper cup of

Coca-Cola from another patient. As she sipped it, she said that it was an egg cream. She wandered around the porch and the dayhall picking cigarette butts up off the floor. She put the cigarette butts in the little bit of Coke remaining. "This is the ultimate drink," she said. "It's vodka. It's schnapps. Cigarette water is chicken soup." She drank it down. Barbara Herbert, who had been watching Miss Frumkin, told her she was disgusting. The two women exchanged insults.

"I'm Brigitte Bardot!" Mrs. Herbert shouted at Miss Frumkin after apparently running out of all the barnyard epithets she knew.

"No, you're not!" Miss Frumkin shouted back.

"God is my father!" Mrs. Herbert yelled.

"I am my mother!" Miss Frumkin screamed, and she marched off stiffly, like a toy soldier that had just been wound up.

After a short period of parading, Miss Frumkin headed for an aqua chair in which a timid-looking elderly woman was sitting. "Excuse me," she said, lifting the frail old lady out of the chair and setting her down on the lap of a patient seated on a nearby sofa. She made herself comfortable in the aqua chair. At one o'clock, after lunch, a therapy aide handed Miss Frumkin two twenty-five-milligram Moban tablets. She swallowed the pills, saying they were eyedrops, and then said, "I was a Buddhist and a born-again Christian, and now I'm trying to get back to my own religion."

Paulette Finestone, who was seated in an adjacent orange chair, said, "Sylvia, you're Jewish, just like me."

Miss Frumkin shrugged, gave Miss Finestone a recipe for mayonnaise in Yiddish, and said that JE 333 was God's phone number. Then, in a strong, clear voice, she sang, "We three kings of Orient are, raising prices of fueling your car." Then she said "Praise the Lord," and, temporarily spent, sprawled sidewise across the aqua chair. A while later, she put the words of what she said was the Thirty-seventh Psalm to the tune of "Desiderata." The words were one part Twenty-third Psalm and three parts gibberish. She then embarked on what sounded like an autobiographical odyssey: "I was born in Brooklyn, where the tree grows. Everyone who is anyone was born in Brooklyn. A tree grows in Brooklyn, so saith Bugs Bunny. If you don't believe me, ask, ask, ask . . . The trouble is, we all moved from Brooklyn to Queens when I was nine. My grandmother may have invented the potato pancake, but I invented the egg cream. I went to the High School of Music and Art. Music and Art became a furniture store, so I went to a private school. My sister Joyce is older than me by — well, if I was born on May 5, 1948, and she was born on September 29, 1942, it must be six years and eight months, no, five years and eight months. Well, whatever, five years, six years, eight years, eight months. I once got an eight on a math test. I even had to wear Joyce's old gym suits and how low can you get? Joyce went to an almost Ivy League college. She's a big shot. Jimmy and Rosalynn are always inviting her to the White House. I've lost a lot of weight at Weight Watchers. I want a lifetime subscription to *Weight Watchers* magazine. Grandma came and lived with us. After Grandma died, four weeks after I turned eighteen, Aunt Lottie came and lived with us. I also had an Aunt Goldie. Doesn't every Jewish family have an Aunt Goldie? Uncle Simon threw me into the water at the University Settlement Camp. The first thing I ever said as a kid was 'See my skinny bones,' because I was Claude Kirchner. I didn't want to play the Wizard of Oz when I was Bob Keeshan. You know what the trouble was? Our cat Gingersnap died. I tortured Gingersnap. I killed the cat. Gingersnap was a middle-aged unicorn." As Miss Frumkin said the word *unicorn,* she paused, got up, and walked toward the mural on the dayhall wall until she was only a few inches away from it — a distance from which she could see it without her glasses. "Is this a nuthouse?" she asked the unicorn in the mural. "Do elephants like peanuts?

I fell into the gap. I don't want to come out. I've been married five times. You want Ringo, I want Paul, and the prince wants me. Elton John is John Yarrow. One thing about Creedmoor, it's like a rainbow. When I leave here, I'm going on a long vacation. Transitional can borrow me, but I always come back. I own the place. My father built it." Stepping over a woman who was sleeping on the floor, she sat down on a vacant chair and said, "I'm the one loser."

While Miss Frumkin was singing her version of "We Three Kings of Orient Are," Transitional Services' clinical coordinator, Peter Orenstein, and a nurse from Transitional Services were listening to her. They had come to the ward to visit Miss Frumkin. She had ignored them. After watching part of her performance in the dayhall, they were troubled by what they had seen, and asked Stephanie Fulton, the treatment-team leader for 043 and 044, to let them read Miss Frumkin's chart. When they had read it, the nurse said sadly to Dr. Sun, who was in the chart room, "She's so out of contact. She's so out of control. How could we have lost so much ground in three days?" Orenstein asked Miss Fulton to please keep him informed about Miss Frumkin's progress. He said that Transitional Services would try to hold her place for a while, in the hope that she would soon be over this crisis. The nurse wrote a note about their visit on Miss Frumkin's record at Transitional Services. "Sylvia appears to be having an acute schizophrenic episode," the note read. "She was extremely bizarre and inappropriate in appearance and her conversation. She made frequent reference to her sister 'Joyce and her White House invitations.' The face was covered with lipstick and her attention span was very short. She apparently is prone to agitated behavior, because there had been numerous seclusion orders written on her chart."

That afternoon, Dr. Sun wrote out an order to discontinue the Moban tablets. Moban wasn't of any use to a patient as agitated as Miss Frumkin, he said later. He prescribed 400 milligrams of Thorazine liquid for Miss Frumkin, to be taken twice a day in 200-milligram doses. He increased the dosage of the Thorazine injections she was to be given as needed for severe agitation, from 50 milligrams every four hours to 75 milligrams every two hours. And he put down on her chart that she should have another skull X ray, an electroencephalogram, and a neurological consultation in Building 40. This order was apparently overlooked: Months went by and Miss Frumkin didn't go to Building 40 for the skull X ray, the EEG, or the neurological consultation.

Later that afternoon, Miss Frumkin had another hostile exchange of words with Barbara Herbert and a fight with Paulette Finestone after she had grabbed a Bible that Miss Finestone was quietly reading; she sang "Big Wide Wonderful World" in a loud voice; and she outtalked everyone else in the ward. "I created the Muppets," she said just before dinner. "I'm the first woman mayor of Hollywood. I lost more weight than anyone else at Weight Watchers. My cat's name was Strawberry Butterscotch McLean. Strawberry is my favorite flavor. I like strawberry ice cream, strawberry shortcake, strawberry anything. Senior day is drawing to a close. I'm going to marry John Travolta." Miss Frumkin splattered a substantial amount of the food she intended to eat for dinner over her already stained clothes. She was distraught early in the evening, but quieted down for a couple of hours after swallowing her 200 milligrams of Thorazine and went to bed. She didn't sleep well. During the night of the nineteenth, the nurse management team was called twice, Miss Frumkin was given two injections of Thorazine, and she spent a good part of the night in the seclusion room, yelling, banging on the door, and keeping the patients in the dormitory awake.

Soon after Miss Frumkin was let out of the seclusion room on the morning of June 20, she hit another woman. She spent most of the day back in the seclusion room, where she was served her lunch and dinner. In the evening, a therapy aide opened the door to the seclusion room to give Miss Frumkin her medication. She took the paper cup containing her Thorazine and raised it to her mouth. Just as she seemed to be about to swallow it, she threw it in the therapy aide's face. The Thorazine hit the therapy aide's right eye, temporarily blinding her. Another therapy aide, who was standing in the corridor behind her, rushed her to a faucet and applied a cold-water compress to her eye. The doctor on call was notified. Miss Frumkin was given an injection of Thorazine and was secluded again. Each time a two-hour seclusion order expired and a therapy aide let her out of the seclusion room, Miss Frumkin attacked the therapy aide and was put back in.

Early on the morning of June 21, both Miss Frumkin and the seclusion room were filthy. Miss Frumkin refused to take a shower. A nurse from the nurse management team and several aides gave Miss Frumkin a shower, put clean underwear, a clean blouse, and a clean pair of black slacks on her, and washed out the seclusion room. Before they had finished cleaning the room, she had attacked several other staff members, and she was put back in the seclusion room. That morning, Dr. Sun increased her daily medication to 600 milligrams of Thorazine — 200 milligrams in the morning, 400 milligrams before going to bed. At noon, Miss Frumkin was let out of seclusion. She ate lunch in the dining room, addressing her three tablemates as Mary Tyler Moore, Jesus Christ, and Barbara Walters. Upon her return to the dayhall, she took her slacks off and tried to hit several other patients, who managed to dodge her. She was put in seclusion for two hours. When she was let out in the evening, she knocked Paulette Finestone's eyeglasses off her nose; Miss Finestone's glasses broke in half. Miss Frumkin spent most of the night of the twenty-first in the seclusion room, and a good part of the next day as well. It often required several people to give her an injection of Thorazine. On the night of the twenty-second, she slept in the seclusion room with the door open. At four-thirty in the morning on June 23, she went into the dormitory and attacked some of the patients who were sleeping there. The women started to scream and run away from her. It took two team members of the staff to put Miss Frumkin back in seclusion.

Later that morning, the nurse on Miss Frumkin's treatment team told Dr. Sun that Miss Frumkin was still highly agitated. The nurse reported that she was refusing to take her oral medication, that she lashed out against those who gave her injections, and that she hit and kicked them so badly that it was all but impossible for them to take her vital signs. The nurse brought Miss Frumkin into Dr. Sun's office. Dr. Sun spoke softly to Miss Frumkin, and she calmly let him remove the three stitches from her head. She was calm for fifteen minutes more, then started to rant and rave and was put back in seclusion. She was in and out of seclusion that day and that night. The doctor on night duty, who came to write a seclusion order on her chart at five-twenty on the morning of the twenty-fourth, after the nurse management team had asked him for one, arrived just as Miss Frumkin was waking up. She told him that it made her miserable not to be able to see anything, and asked him if she could have her eyeglasses. On the off chance that she might settle down if she was given her glasses, the doctor asked a therapy aide to get them out of the private-clothing room for her. She put the glasses on. A few minutes later, she threw them on the floor and ran down the hallway, banging on the doors, grabbing things off desks and throwing them on the floor, and hitting patients and staff members. She was put back into seclusion. The doctor who had given her the eyeglasses suggested that Dr. Sun review Miss Frumkin's medication when he came to work on Monday morning, the twenty-sixth.

There was no improvement in Miss Frumkin's behavior on the twenty-fifth or the twenty-sixth. She refused a good deal of her oral medication, took other patients' belongings, and attempted to kick and bite the staff members who tried to stop her or gave her injections. On the twenty-sixth, Dr. Sun increased her medication to 900 milligrams of Thorazine. On the twenty-seventh, Miss Frumkin tried to take Barbara Herbert's handbag. Mrs. Herbert bit her on the right cheek and on her back. The bites were cleaned with hydrogen peroxide, and Miss Frumkin was given a tetanus shot. On the twenty-seventh, Dr. Sun increased her Thorazine to 1200 milligrams a day. On the twenty-ninth, he increased it to 1500 milligrams — 500 milligrams three times a day. She was still hyperactive, was still abusive toward patients and staff, and still spent a good deal of time in the seclusion room. On the evening of June 29, a licensed practical nurse came to the seclusion room to give her 500 milligrams of liquid Thorazine. The nurse was an attractive West Indian. Miss Frumkin called her Diahann Carroll, told her she didn't like the way she sang, ordered her to "get out of my face," and grabbed the medication and threw it at her, spilling it all over her blouse. She was put back into seclusion. By June 29, there were fifty seclusion orders on her chart.

Friday, June 30, was the first day since her admission to Creedmoor, two weeks earlier, that Miss Frumkin was able to stay out of the seclusion room for twenty-four hours straight. On the morning of the thirtieth, she was wearing a dirty white blouse, a pair of size-18 purple slacks (she insisted that they were size 11), a blue-and-white saddle shoe on her right foot, and a brown pump on her left foot. She was carrying two handbags — her own and one that had been given to her by Barbara Herbert. She gave Mrs. Herbert's pocketbook away to the first person who asked her for it. She was also wearing Mrs. Herbert's wedding band. She said that Mrs. Herbert had given her the handbag and the wedding band because Mrs. Herbert was sorry she had bitten her so badly three days earlier. Miss Frumkin's fingernails were painted with a silvery-blue shade of nail polish. The day was hot. At ten o'clock, Miss Frumkin was sitting on a sofa with a pretty young woman named Eileen O'Reilly, who had been admitted to Creedmoor three days after Miss Frumkin with what appeared to be a drug-induced psychosis. Miss O'Reilly was a college student. In April, she had been admitted to Creedmoor and discharged after a week. In May, she had again been admitted and discharged after a week. When she returned to Creedmoor in June, her delusions had cleared up quickly on antipsychotic medication; most of the drug addicts who are admitted to Creedmoor are symptom-free after a few days of treatment. Miss O'Reilly, who had never been hospitalized before 1978, had decided to stay at the hospital for a while to try to work out some of the problems that had brought her to Creedmoor three times in three months. A psychologist newly hired for 043 and 044 had promised to work with her several hours a week. Meanwhile, Miss O'Reilly had found Clearview boring and depressing. She was an intelligent young woman and a good listener. She had soon decided that Miss Frumkin was the least boring patient in Clearview (it was Miss O'Reilly who had called her "the greatest show on earth") and the most fun to listen to and to observe, perhaps because Miss Frumkin carried everything to such extremes: She talked too much, she talked too fast, she moved like a whirling dervish, and she could always be counted on to do something outlandish. Ten minutes earlier, when one of the male patients had asked Miss Frumkin for some of the water she was drinking from a paper cup, she had poured the water that remained in the cup over his head. "You wanted water, now you got water," she had told him.

Miss O'Reilly looked at Miss Frumkin's pocketbook and said that it was too full. Since there was nothing better to do in the ward, she offered to help her clean it out. Miss Frumkin looked doubtful, but when Miss O'Reilly got up and returned with a wastebasket she had found in a corner of the dayhall, Miss Frumkin allowed her to open the pocketbook, turn it upside down, and spill the contents on the sofa between them. The two women went through all the items that had been in the pocketbook. Miss O'Reilly was allowed to put a rusty paper clip, a candy-bar wrapper, a bobby pin that was bent out of shape, a straw with lipstick marks at both ends, and a knotted piece of white satin ribbon into the wastebasket. Miss Frumkin watched her without comment. When Miss O'Reilly threw a couple of dozen cigarette butts in the wastebasket, Miss Frumkin said, "I only smoke when I'm sick. I'm allergic to cigarette smoke when I'm well, and I hate cigarettes then." When Miss O'Reilly riffled through a number of pages torn from magazines, and prepared to crumple them and toss them into the wastebasket, Miss Frumkin looked at a page with a shampoo ad that included a picture of a beautiful blond woman. She said that the woman resembled her sister, Joyce. When Miss O'Reilly put a broken pencil in the wastebasket, Miss Frumkin said she had terrible handwriting when she was sick but almost legible handwriting when she was well. An earring with a broken clip, a ring that was missing six out of seven fake stones, and twelve cherry pits were relegated to the wastebasket. When Miss O'Reilly tried to throw out a batch of cents-off coupons clipped from newspapers and magazines, Miss Frumkin called a halt to the pocketbook-cleaning operation. "My mother saves coupons," she said, stuffing dollar-off cigarette coupons, ten-cents-off dog-food coupons, and seven-cents-off tuna-fish coupons back into her bag. "My parents are very cheap," she said. Back into her bag also went a well-worn prayer book, a real-estate brochure, a small notebook, a frazzled toothbrush, a ball-point pen, a calorie book, three paperback books, a bankbook, four used-up tubes of lipstick, and a broken mirror.

Miss O'Reilly had grounds privileges and some money. She told Miss Frumkin that she was going out to a delicatessen on Hillside Avenue for a sandwich and a soda. Miss Frumkin had no money, but she asked Miss O'Reilly to bring her a container of honey-flavored yogurt from the delicatessen. She promised to pay Miss O'Reilly back. When Miss O'Reilly returned with the yogurt, Miss Frumkin rummaged through her bag looking for a spoon. She seemed to be aware that there was no spoon in the bag, but she insisted on rummaging anyway. Finding no spoon, she took out her toothbrush and began to eat the yogurt with the toothbrush. Miss O'Reilly laughed at her. Miss Frumkin didn't seem to mind. "They laughed at Bell and they laughed at Edison," she said, throwing the toothbrush into the wastebasket. She finished eating the yogurt with her fingers.

"I'm a doctor, you know," she told Miss O'Reilly. "I don't have a diploma, but I'm a doctor. I'm glad to be a mental patient, because it taught me how to be humble. I use Cover Girl creamy natural makeup. Oral Roberts has been here to visit me. My sister's name is Joyce Frumkin, and I like her. My father is five feet two inches, my mother is five feet three inches. They're like Napoleon and Josephine, and they're shrinking. Joyce is five-two. I'm only five foot four and I'm the tallest one in my family. This place is where *Mad* magazine is published. The Nixons make Noxon metal polish. When I was a little girl, I used to sit and tell stories to myself. When I was older, I turned off the sound on the TV set and made up dialogue to go with the shows I watched. The people in Creedmoor are Hobbits. I dictated the Hobbit stories to Tolkien, and he took them all down. I'm the Hobbit. Ask John Denver. He told me I was. I'm the only person who ever got Ringo Starr angry. All the trouble started when my father decided to move from Brooklyn to Queens when I was seven. I went to the eleventh grade twice — once at Music and Art, a public school for gifted musicians and artists, and once at a private school. Jesus told me he was born nineteen hundred and seventy-three years ago. He's my best friend. I call him J.C. I was unhappy at school because I was bad in gym. I was unhappy at school because I was only friendly with the underdogs. I had a car accident when I was fifteen. After that, my mother said, my eyes were never the same. My mother's the real dictator. My grandmother left me all her money. I was named for my grandfather Saul, who died five years before I was born. He was born on Easter Sunday. I'm a week pregnant. I have schizophrenia — cancer of the nerves. My body is overcrowded with nerves. This is going to win me the Nobel Prize for medicine. I don't consider myself schizophrenic anymore. There's no such thing as schizophrenia, there's only mental telepathy. I once had a friend named Camilla Costello. She was Abbott and Costello's daughter. She said to me, 'You know, Sylvia, I have a lot of friends, but you're my best friend.' I'm working here. I'm an intern at Creedmoor. I'm in the Pentecostal Church, but I'm thinking of changing my religion. I have a dog at home. I love instant oatmeal. When you have Jesus, you don't need a diet. Mick Jagger wants to marry me. I want to get out the revolving door. With Jesus Christ, anything is possible. I used to hit my mother. It was the hyperactivity from all the cookies I ate. I'm the personification of Casper the Friendly Ghost. I used to go outside asking the other kids to be my friend when I was little. California's the most beautiful state in the Union. I've been there once, by television. My name is Jack Warden, and I'm an actress."

Miss Frumkin, who had been alternately tugging on her bangs and twiddling with the lace on her saddle shoe, got angry with two female patients who approached the sofa on which she and Miss O'Reilly were seated and eavesdropped on her conversation. She took off her brown pump and threw it at one of them. She got up off the sofa and tried to take the belt off the other patient's dress, saying she needed it as a hair band. The two interlopers moved elsewhere. Miss Frumkin retrieved her pump, sat down, and asked Miss O'Reilly to write a letter for her. She reached into her bag and gave Miss O'Reilly her notebook and her ball-point pen. "Take a letter," she said, as if she were accustomed to dictating her correspondence every day. "To Dr. Sun from Sylvia Frumkin," she began. "Dear Dr. Sun: The above-named patient being of legal age and of sound mind and body does hereby request her discharge as of three days from the above date. If proper action on this matter is not taken, the above-named will begin legal proceedings against this hospital. Yours truly, with love, Sylvia." She told Miss O'Reilly to date the letter June 29, although, she said, she knew that it was June 30. She told her she was doing this because the hospital had seventy-two hours in which to reply to her letter and she didn't feel like waiting more than forty-eight hours. A few seconds later, she told Miss O'Reilly to tear up the letter. "I think I'd be certified on a two-physicians certificate, and I don't feel like putting it to the test," she explained. "I'm better off as a voluntary patient. Besides, it's comfortable here. We don't have to do many things we don't want to do, and Dr. Sun is defending me against the forces of evil. Take another letter. This one is for Keith Amerigo, Esquire, attendant, from Sylvia Frumkin. Subject: love and marriage. Dear Sir: When a woman as I am feels as she does about a man such as you are, there is no other word to say but that she deeply mourns her love for you and has abandoned all others because she is your only one and you are her only one. With love, Future."

"Sylvia, Amerigo's as queer as a three-dollar bill," Miss O'Reilly said. Miss Frumkin looked at Miss O'Reilly skeptically.

A patient seated nearby commented sarcastically on Miss Frumkin's mismatched shoes. "It's a new style I've invented," she said. "Someday, it will make me famous." Miss Frumkin sat in silence briefly. "I guess wearing two different shoes is going overboard," she told Miss O'Reilly. "I was just doing it to entertain some people." She said she was going to the clothing room to look for either a second blue-and-white saddle shoe or a second brown pump. She returned ten minutes later, barefoot and carrying a pair of gold sandals, and sat down next to Miss O'Reilly. It was time for her to take her midday dose of liquid Thorazine.

When a nurse handed her the 500 milligrams in a paper cup, she said she didn't want to swallow it. Miss O'Reilly urged her to take it. Miss Frumkin did. She then got angry at Miss O'Reilly for making her take her medicine, and wouldn't speak to her for the rest of the day.

⁂

In 1978, 2759 people were admitted to Creedmoor. The median length of stay was thirty-eight days. Of these admissions, 1853 — sixty-seven percent — were people who, like Sylvia Frumkin, had been at Creedmoor previously. While Thorazine and other antipsychotic drugs have reduced New York State's mental-hospital population by approximately seventy-three percent since they were first tested on a grand scale, in 1954, there is a core of chronic mental patients who have not been permanently helped by these drugs. Many of those released in the 1950s, 1960s, and 1970s have had to be readmitted. Some return to the hospital every five or ten years. The pre-Thorazine pattern of first admissions that became last admissions because the patients stayed in the hospitals until they died has largely given way to a pattern of multiple admissions. In 1976, Hermine Plotnick had reviewed the admissions histories of forty-one patients admitted to the Clearview unit in one month. She had learned that thirty-eight of the forty-one were readmissions, and that two of the remaining three patients had come from Hillside. Only one patient seemed, from the record, not to have had prior psychiatric treatment. Many families in the middle-income and upper-middle-income sections of the Clearview catchment area, which is the most prosperous catchment area in Queens, did not resort to state hospitals for their relatives until they had spent tens of thousands of dollars on private psychiatrists and private hospitals, and for this reason Clearview's patients often came in with more advanced cases of mental illness than patients in other units.

Nevertheless, few patients came to the hospital as disturbed as Sylvia Frumkin was on June 16, 1978, and most patients, whatever their state upon admission, settled down within forty-eight hours on oral medication and were released without ever receiving an injection, seeing the inside of a seclusion room, or meeting a member of the nurse management team. Two people were admitted to Clearview on June 16, 1978 — Miss Frumkin and a man named Stephen Lawton. Mr. Lawton was discharged three days later.

For the first two weeks after her admission, Miss Frumkin was the most troublesome patient in wards 043 and 044. The fact that she was Clearview's most difficult "management problem" was evident from the number of seclusion orders on her chart, from her medication record, from the progress notes that the therapy aides on each shift were required to make every day for the first few days of a patient's stay and at least once a week (more often, if necessary) in subsequent weeks, and from the entries in the ward's communication book. The communication book was a bound notebook kept on the long table in the chart room, in which staff members were supposed to record pertinent happenings in the ward, primarily for the benefit of the staff on the other shifts and for staff members returning from days off, leaves, and vacations. If a patient had to have a blood-sugar measurement on an empty stomach at nine o'clock on a Wednesday morning, a therapy aide on the Tuesday day shift would make a note of it in the communication book, so that the Wednesday-morning shift would make sure that the patient wasn't given breakfast. When evening- and night-shift employees found shortages of ward supplies, they listed the supplies they needed in the communication book, so that the day-shift staff could order the missing blankets and mops and other items; the storehouse was open only in the daytime.

A Clearview patient who had grounds privileges had wandered away from Creedmoor on June 14, 1978. When word got back to the hospital on June 20 that her body had been found in the Hudson River, Stephanie Fulton wrote in the communication book, "We received news today that Jeanne Knight died this morning. Some pts. seem to know about this. Please let them talk about it if they need to. If you are aware of pts. like Sean Flint that were close to her, please try and spend time with them because they will probably take the news badly and need some support. Thank you. Stephanie." Many entries in the communication book concerned patient escapes — so that the staff of subsequent shifts would know for the count made at all three changes of shift that any patients who had escaped were already missing — and behavior problems, to alert subsequent shifts to those patients requiring special observation and attention. The patient whose name appeared in the communication book most frequently between June 16 and June 30 was Sylvia Frumkin. Two typical entries read: "6-18-78. Morning Report, 12–8. Sylvia Frumkin became very agitated at 1 A.M. NMT [nurse management team] called. Dr. Mohan Dutt ordered seclusion. Pt. talked all night"; and "6-29-78. Morning Report, 12–8. Frumkin remains very agitated and abusive. Pt. is in seclusion."

On June 30, the therapy aide who did the report for the night shift wrote in the communication book, "Patients quiet, apparently comfortable. Sylvia Frumkin created no problems." Miss Frumkin had been so difficult for so long that it was news that she was no longer news.

II

Disappearing Incidents

Five

Between June 30 and July 6, Miss Frumkin seemed to take a turn for the better — or, at least, for the quieter. She wasn't put in seclusion. She wasn't given any Thorazine injections for agitation. She willingly swallowed 500 milligrams of liquid Thorazine three times a day. Dr. Sun had left for a two-week vacation on July 3 without changing this dose, which he had raised her to on June 29. During the first week of July, Miss Frumkin still expressed a number of delusions: "I'm a Jewish mental-patient detective," she insisted on July 1. She also wore odd costumes: On July 2, she was wearing a blouse draped over one shoulder and tied around her neck by the sleeves, and had wrapped herself up in a pink blanket. When her father came to visit her on July 3, she didn't hit him (as she had done once in June) or ignore him (as she had done on several occasions in June). He had brought her some of the many things she had asked him for the previous day, when she had called home — some Sensodyne toothpaste and a Sensodyne toothbrush (she said that she had sensitive teeth), some Cepacol mouthwash, a bar of Ivory soap (the only kind, she said, she could use on her sensitive skin), and a spare pair of eyeglasses, which the Frumkins kept at home for her.

When Mr. Frumkin took the things he had brought from home out of a shopping bag, his daughter examined them, berated him for the items she had requested that he had failed to bring her — a can of apricot nectar, a bag of popcorn, a nail clipper — and then thanked him, in her fashion, for the glasses. "Oh, you brought my glasses," she said, putting them on. She lost the toothpaste, the soap, and the mouthwash within twenty-four hours. She kept the glasses and seemed grateful that she could see clearly after two and a half weeks in a myopic haze. On July 4, she hit Paulette Finestone with her pocketbook, but in general she was less combative. On July 5, she asked to see Dr. Shamaldaree Batra, who was handling Dr. Sun's patients during his vacation. She told him she wanted to go off all medication, and threatened to sue him for malpractice when he didn't consent. On July 6, when Dr. Batra was walking through the women's dayhall, Miss Frumkin loped over to him and said, "Sweet Dr. Batra, why don't you go into my office and we'll make love?" Dr. Batra smiled and kept on walking. When Hermine Plotnick was making her daily rounds on the sixth, she noticed that Miss Frumkin was still "talking schizophrenia," as she put it, but she thought that the medication was beginning to take hold.

On the morning of Friday, July 7, Miss Frumkin got up and dressed herself in a flowered nylon half-slip, a bra, a long-sleeved navy-blue T-shirt, and a pair of high-heeled gold sandals. She put on her glasses and tied a kerchief around her hair. She ate breakfast and refused her morning medication. Her mood seemed more defiant than it had been in the past week, and the therapy aides didn't criticize her attire. At eight-thirty, the ward cleaner wanted to mop the women's dayhall. It was a warm, bright day. Miss Frumkin and the other women in the dayhall who didn't have grounds privileges were told to go out on the porch. A nurse came out to the porch a few minutes later with injections for Miss Frumkin (because she had refused her oral medication) and

Barbara Herbert, who had been obstreperous all morning. Miss Frumkin called the nurse "the pusher" and bent over reluctantly to get her Thorazine injection. She bled slightly where the needle had been inserted. "They struck blood, which proves I'm Jesus Christ," she said, and she invited the others on the porch to drink her blood. Mrs. Herbert called her a pig. While the floor of the dayhall was drying, Hiroku Izutsu sang a song to the tune of "Alouette":

> Medication, Creedmoor medication,
> Medication, the pills we love to pop.
> First you take a Stelazine, then you take a Thorazine,
> Mellaril, Elavil,
> Tofranil, what a thrill!
> Oh —
> Medication, Creedmoor medication,
> Medication, the pills we love to pop.

A few of the women laughed appreciatively. Miss Frumkin appeared to be envious of Miss Izutsu's cleverness and of the attention she had received while she sang. She took a banana out of her pocketbook, ate it, used the banana peel to wipe off her glasses, seemed pleased when someone said, "Sylvia, you're too much," threw the banana peel on the floor, and recited a poem called "Supreme Egotism," which she said she had just written.

> She thinks that she
> Has the most
> Colorful mind in
> The whole star-
> Studded universe,
> But,
> Confidentially,
> I have.

After reciting the poem, she said "That poem means I am the best," and sat down. She looked pleased with herself for having regained center stage.

"Sylvia, why don't you ever give your mouth a rest?" one of the other patients said.

"I've got to stay here with my children," Miss Frumkin answered. "They are my children. I've been here long enough to be Mother Goose to them."

By nine o'clock the dayhall floor was dry, and the patients on the porch were told they could go back inside. Miss Frumkin ran into the women's dayhall, saw that the door leading to 044, the men's ward, was open, ran down the corridor to the men's dayhall, said, in passing, to a therapy aide in 044, "I'm Jack Warden and I'm making a movie and I want to see the doctor," and ran through an open door that led from the 044 dayhall to the chart room, where the patients' records were kept. Diana Bancroft, a psychologist who had started work in the Clearview unit a week earlier, was standing in the doorway and heard what Miss Frumkin had said to the therapy aide as she breezed by. Miss Bancroft followed Miss Frumkin into the chart room and invited her to come to her office, hoping she could calm her down. Miss Frumkin ignored Miss Bancroft and sailed through the chart room. There she saw Dr. Batra, and immediately demanded to go to Jewish services. The Frumkins are Jewish and attend services at their temple two or three times a year — on Rosh Hashanah and on Yom Kippur. When Miss Frumkin was not in Creedmoor, she accompanied her parents to temple on these holy days. When she was in Creedmoor, she usually attended Jewish services held every Friday morning in the Assembly Hall, a building that was about a five-minute walk from Building N/4. Each Friday, the rabbi led a congregation of about fifty or sixty white, black, and Hispanic Catholics, Protestants, and Jews in prayer. He spoke from nine-forty-five to ten. His sermon was followed by refreshments provided by various religious and service organizations in Queens. When Miss Frumkin considered herself Jewish, she went to Jewish services faithfully and took notes on the rabbi's sermons. When, periodically, she considered herself a Hebrew-Christian, she went to the Jewish services regularly, mainly for the sandwiches, fruit punch, and cake, and also went to church. When, periodically, she considered herself a born-again Christian, she skipped Jewish services, tore up her notes on the rabbi's sermons, and went to church more often.

When Miss Frumkin burst into the chart room on July 7, Dr. Batra was alone there, writing in a patient's chart. He kept on writing as if he hadn't heard her. "Mental patients have constitutional rights, and I demand that you let me out immediately to go to Jewish services!" Miss Frumkin shouted at him.

Dr. Batra tapped his pen on the table.

"Dr. Batra, if you don't stop tapping your pen, I'll take it away from you!" Miss Frumkin shouted even louder. "Jewish services start at nine-fifteen in the Assembly Hall, and you're making me late!"

Dr. Batra looked up at Miss Frumkin and said, "You want to go to Jewish services? Go ahead." He told Miss Bancroft, who was standing just outside the chart room, to see to it that Miss Frumkin was let out of the ward. Miss Bancroft was stunned. She knew that Miss Frumkin didn't have grounds privileges, and she didn't believe her to be in any condition to go to Jewish services by herself. Two of the things that a treatment team — the psychiatrist, psychologist, social worker, nurse, and therapy aide who work most closely with a patient and who, in theory, jointly decide upon a course of treatment — was supposed to consider before letting a patient out of a locked ward unescorted were the patient's state of mind and state of dress. In Miss Bancroft's opinion, Miss Frumkin's attire that morning — blue T-shirt, flowered half-slip, and high-heeled gold sandals — was altogether inappropriate, and so was her behavior. Like a number of other psychiatrists at Creedmoor, Dr. Batra paid lip service to the concept of the treatment team but often neglected to consult the other team members. Stephanie Fulton, Miss Frumkin's treatment-team leader, had not yet shown up for work (she was often late), but several other members of the team were there. Dr. Batra did not consult them. Nor did he write on the doctor's order sheet in Miss Frumkin's chart that he had given her permission to attend Jewish services — another required procedure.

Miss Frumkin walked quickly to the Assembly Hall. The rabbi, who had known her and her family for years, was startled by her clothes and by her behavior. She kept interrupting his sermon, and after it was over, and he had turned on a tape of "Milk and Honey" and other theater music with a Jewish theme, she tried to convert him to Christianity. Miss Frumkin gulped down three cups of punch and ate two bologna sandwiches and several cupcakes. A volunteer worker who was helping to serve the refreshments, a woman who had also known Miss Frumkin and her family for years, suggested to her that she return to the ward and put a skirt on. Miss Frumkin ignored her. She left the Assembly Hall, but instead of going back to N/4 she walked a short distance to one of the buildings Transitional Services operated on the Creedmoor grounds, and barged into the office of Peter Orenstein, Transitional's clinical coordinator. She told him she wanted Transitional Services to take her back immediately. Orenstein was upset by the way Miss Frumkin looked and sounded. He asked her who had let her out of the ward. When she told him, he telephoned Dr. Batra, informed him of Miss Frumkin's whereabouts, and said that she appeared to be agitated. Dr. Batra called Creedmoor's Safety Department, and asked Safety to pick Miss Frumkin up at Transitional Services and bring her back to Clearview.

By then it was ten-fifteen, and Stephanie Fulton was at work. Soon after her arrival, Diana Bancroft, who had been watching the clock and worrying, told her the circumstances of Miss Frumkin's departure from the ward. Miss Fulton was furious: The team hadn't even met to consider giving Miss Frumkin grounds privileges, because she wasn't ready for this first small step, and here was a doctor — not even the patient's regular doctor — exposing her to possible harm. While Miss Fulton telephoned Mrs. Plotnick to tell her what Dr. Batra had done, Miss Bancroft decided to express her anger by writing a note in Miss Frumkin's chart saying that Dr. Batra had let Miss Frumkin out of the ward against her better judgment and that Miss Frumkin hadn't returned. A few minutes later, Dr. Batra appeared and told Miss Bancroft and Miss Fulton that Miss Frumkin was on her way back to the ward. The two women notified Mrs. Plotnick that Miss Frumkin was all right, and resumed the day's work.

Two safety officers went to Transitional Services and escorted Miss Frumkin back to Clearview's central corridor. To her pleasant surprise, they didn't take her back into the ward but left her just outside the locked door leading to 043 and 044. She waited a few minutes, to be sure they had gone, and then took off again. This time, she left the hospital grounds. She walked through the unlocked gate nearest N/4 onto Hillside Avenue, took a quick inventory of the contents of her handbag, found her bankbook, and went to her bank, a few blocks down Hillside Avenue, where she had the interest for the quarterly period that had ended on June 30 entered in her bankbook. Her bank balance was about two hundred dollars. She then continued to walk down Hillside Avenue.

Around three o'clock in the afternoon, Miss Bancroft noticed that Miss Frumkin was not in the ward. She went to ask Miss Fulton and Dr. Batra where she was. Miss Fulton hadn't seen her all day. Dr. Batra hadn't seen her since he let her leave for Jewish services in the morning. He didn't appear to be concerned that she was missing. "She'll come back," he said. At three-thirty, Dr. Batra called the Safety Department to report that Miss Frumkin was missing. "She probably went home," he told Miss Fulton and Miss Bancroft, and then he telephoned the Frumkins to ask if she was there. Many patients who wander off from Creedmoor do go home. Miss Frumkin hadn't gone home, and her parents were distressed to learn that a doctor had let a young woman in her condition venture out of the building alone. Miss Fulton and a therapy aide got into Miss Fulton's car and drove up and down the streets surrounding Creedmoor looking for her. They didn't find her.

Miss Frumkin was found by two policemen from a neighboring precinct at ten past eight that evening. She was still wearing a kerchief on her head, gold sandals on her feet, and a half-slip. She was no longer wearing a T-shirt, and her bra was open. Four months later, in November, she recalled that she had had a lovely afternoon. She had browsed in some of the stores near her bank. She had walked to the Happy Robin, an inexpensive restaurant on Hillside Avenue that served meals cafeteria-style. She had often eaten at the Happy Robin with her parents. She had asked a woman behind the counter for a glass of water and, when the woman gave her the water, had said to her, "Smile. You're on *Candid Camera.*" She knew that there were sliced raw onions as well as salt and pepper and other condiments at the Happy Robin, so she had sat down at a table and eaten a few free onions. "I do crazy things when I'm sick, and then I don't know why when I'm well," she said that November. When the policemen picked Miss Frumkin up on Hillside Avenue in her state of semi-undress, she went with them peaceably. She also remembered that she had been having a fantasy about being in the police department on that warm July day. She knew that policemen sometimes had nicknames — she had learned that from seeing a movie called *The Super Cops* on television, in which two policemen were known as Batman and Robin. She had told the policemen that her nickname was the Pink Streak. "Oh, yeah, I've heard of you," she remembered one of them telling her as they escorted her back to Clearview.

When the police returned Miss Frumkin to Clearview, a therapy aide on the evening shift found her extremely hyperactive and confused. She was placed in a locked seclusion room for a short time and was given some food and then her evening medication — 500 milligrams of Thorazine. The doctor on night duty who was called to Clearview to examine Miss Frumkin found her in good physical condition. She fell asleep around ten o'clock in an unlocked seclusion room. By that time, the therapy aide had called Mrs. Plotnick and the Frumkins. Harriet Frumkin didn't seem surprised to learn that her almost topless daughter was back in the hospital without having been molested. "That girl has more lives than a cat," she said.

Six

Voluntary patients who take off from Creedmoor, as Miss Frumkin did on July 7, 1978, are said to have gone on a leave without consent, or LWOC. If they succeed in staying away from the hospital for three days, they are discharged. The official reasoning behind the discharge is that the state is required by law to reply within seventy-two hours to a voluntary patient's written request for release, and that a patient's departure is considered the equivalent of such a letter. In the absence of the patient, the state cannot turn down the patient's request for release, because in order to do so it must have two physicians certify the patient — a procedure mandated by the New York State Mental Hygiene Law. Therefore, the regulations hold, the patient is to be discharged. People who are at Creedmoor involuntarily — as fewer than a third of the patients were in 1978 — are officially said to have escaped if they decamp. If they manage to stay away, they are discharged when the term of their commitment expires; forensic patients — those who have been accused of a crime and found unfit to stand trial because of mental disease or defect, or those who have been tried and acquitted for the same reason — are the only exception.

In 1978, when a patient at Creedmoor was discovered to have gone on an LWOC or to have escaped, a New York State Office of Mental Health Form 147 — an incident report — was supposed to be filled out in triplicate. Form 147 was supposed to be used for other types of incidents as well. An incident report was supposed to be filled out at Creedmoor, or any of the state's other mental hospitals, when, for instance, a patient was injured accidentally by himself or others; when a patient fought with or assaulted another patient; when a patient assaulted a visitor; when a patient assaulted a member of the staff; when a staff member was accused of abusing a patient; when a patient attempted to commit suicide, as five patients in the Clearview unit did in 1978, or succeeded in committing suicide, as Lloyd Colvin did on February 1, 1979; or when a patient died suddenly, as Alexander Morton did after a fight with another patient, on October 13, 1978. (According to the autopsy, Morton's death resulted from a heart attack.)

An incident report was also supposed to be filled out when a patient was improperly medicated. The potential hazard of medication errors had been demonstrated two years earlier. On Saturday, October 9, 1976, four of Clearview's patients suffered grand-mal seizures; one of the four, an elderly man, died that afternoon. Mrs. Plotnick and one of her treatment-team leaders were able to reconstruct what had apparently happened. The four patients who had had the seizures were all on heavy doses of liquid Thorazine. Liquid Thorazine comes in two concentrations — 30 milligrams to the milliliter and 100 milligrams to the milliliter. Creedmoor's pharmacy had routinely been carrying the lighter concentration and had only recently begun to stock the heavier one. The drug company that manufactures Thorazine puts the different concentrations in bottles that vary in size, in the color of their labels, and in the color of their rubber droppers. When Mrs. Plotnick and the treatment-team leader interviewed the ward's medication-certified therapy aides individually and asked each to pour a certain dose of Thorazine, they watched with horror as one therapy aide poured the Thorazine from the wrong bottle — from a bottle containing the 100-milligram concentrate. The four patients had presumably been given more than three times their prescribed doses. Creedmoor's pharmacy immediately went back to stocking Thorazine in only the lighter concentration.

According to Clearview's records, which were kept by the unit's medical nurse, Clearview's patients were involved in 160 incidents of all types in 1978. Mrs. Plotnick estimates that there were actually almost six times that number, or roughly 900. Some incidents were never reported on a Form 147 because the patients involved were unable or unwilling to report them, no staff member saw them, and any patients who saw them were unable or afraid to report them. On July 29, 1978, Nicholas Taliaferro, a manic-depressive who had been in and out of Creedmoor, forced a Spanish-speaking woman, who had been brought to the hospital suffering from a severe case of postpartum depression, into an act of fellatio in the women's dayhall. The young woman screamed after the sexual assault. She then went into a near-catatonic state that lasted for several days, until she was discharged to her husband, who sent her and their new baby home to her family in Nicaragua. In 1978, Taliaferro had sexual intercourse with a number of women in the Clearview unit, some of whom consented, some of whom lacked the capacity for consenting. Only one of these sexual escapades was the subject of an incident report, and that one was recorded because two staff members were injured when they went into the men's bathroom to separate Taliaferro and his willing partner. The extent of Taliaferro's sex life at Clearview became more apparent when it was discovered, in January of 1979, that he had gonorrhea. Clearview's nurses gave him 4,800,000 units of penicillin. They gave identical doses of penicillin to ten women patients whom they suspected of having been exposed to the gonococcus bacteria by Taliaferro, and whom the staff considered unreliable informants of their sexual liaisons. A number of Clearview's therapy aides disapprove of the frequent examples of "sexual acting out" that they can't help seeing, and are reluctant to fill out incident reports on a subject they find so unsavory.

A great many other incidents, of a less lurid nature, were also not recorded, either because the staff — particularly the therapy aides, who had to write up most of the description on the front of a Form 147 — didn't consider them serious enough, or because they were too busy to fill forms out, or both. The number of reported assaults on patients by other patients (thirty-four) and fights between patients (eighteen) were also well below the actual number of assaults and fights that took place. Many of these incidents were written up only because patients had to be sent out of the ward for medical treatment.

According to Clearview's records, there were thirteen cases of assault on the staff by patients in 1978. Mrs. Plotnick estimates that there were twenty times that many. It was the exceptional day at Clearview when twenty-four hours went by without several patients slapping, kicking, scratching, pushing, or biting therapy aides or throwing chairs, mops, or cigarette urns at them. (Therapy aides were the most likely targets, because they outnumbered all other employees and had the most frequent contact with patients.) Most of these assaults went unreported because they were minor and because the therapy aides, a number of whom were barely literate, disliked paperwork. Another reason that some therapy aides didn't write up minor assaults was that they felt sympathy for their assailants; they believed that the patients wouldn't have lashed out at them if the patients had not been mentally disturbed, and they accepted minor incidents as an occupational hazard. Some of the attendants were less sympathetic to patients; indeed, it seemed to Mrs. Plotnick and the treatment-team leaders that about five percent of

Clearview's therapy aides provoked attacks from the patients by their own hostile attitudes, and received about ninety-five percent of the minor injuries. These therapy aides often didn't fill out incident reports, either, because in most cases it did them no good. Mental patients, by reason of their being mental patients, often could not be held responsible for their acts.

Easily the most contentious category of incidents at Creedmoor is abuse of patients by staff members. There were two reported cases of alleged abuse of patients in the Clearview unit in 1978. The first involved a therapy aide named Paul Torres, who pummeled a patient named Marshall Lopez after Lopez threw a chair at him and then punched him. When the hospital tried to dismiss Torres, the therapy aides' union, the Civil Service Employees Association, took the case to arbitration. The arbitrator decided that the hospital had failed to prove its case conclusively but that Torres was "wanting in professional judgment." He ordered Torres returned to his job, with a penalty of six weeks' suspension without pay.

The second case still rankles Mrs. Plotnick. It is the only one she has ever lost before an arbitrator, and involved a therapy aide named Crystal Chamberlin and a fifty-year-old manic-depressive patient named Josephine Sandusky. On May 29, 1978, according to a licensed practical nurse who witnessed the incident, Miss Sandusky, after refusing to take a pill that had been prescribed for her, emptied a paper cup filled with water on Miss Chamberlin's wig. Miss Chamberlin, according to the nurse, "then pushed the patient to the wall several times, banged the patient's head against the wall, pushed the patient to the floor, banged her head against the floor several times, and kicked the patient on the arms." Two other therapy aides were in the room at the time the incident occurred. After the incident, a doctor treated Miss Sandusky for a small bruise and a swelling on the left side of her scalp, and a small laceration on her right elbow. The abuse of patients by staff members is particularly abhorrent to Mrs. Plotnick. She looks upon mental patients as among the most defenseless human beings, and feels that at a minimum a hospital should ease their lot and see that they are not abused by the staff. After an investigation, the hospital suspended Miss Chamberlin without pay and notified her that she would be dismissed — a move that, in practical terms, meant that the case would be taken to arbitration.

Therapy aides tend to hold a united front against the hospital management in disciplinary matters, apparently on the theory that any one of them could get into trouble and need supporting witnesses someday, and because they are dependent on each other for help in handling the patients in the ward. In this instance, though, Mrs. Plotnick thought the hospital would win, because the two therapy aides had said enough when questioned on the day of the incident to make her believe that they would corroborate the nurse's testimony. At the arbitration hearing, conducted at the offices of the American Arbitration Association, in Manhattan, Miss Chamberlin denied having hit or kicked Miss Sandusky. The nurse who had witnessed the incident testified that she had. The two therapy aides who had also been in the room did not corroborate the nurse's testimony against Miss Chamberlin. One testified, according to the arbitrator's report, that she had seen Miss Chamberlin and Miss Sandusky "holding arms" but that she "saw no blows and heard no screams or yelling," noting that "there was a great deal of noise in that area." The other therapy aide, according to the arbitrator's report, explained that her vision had been "somewhat impaired by a couch." After hearing the conflicting testimony, the arbitrator ruled that the hospital had failed to prove that Miss Chamberlin was guilty, and that she should be returned to work with full back pay; any mention of the incident was to be removed from her personnel file.

Despite the difficulty of proving physical abuse of patients, Mrs. Plotnick does not believe that it is frequent. She thinks that genuine sadists would find a less arduous way of satisfying their desire to hurt people than working for low wages in conditions as taxing as those at Creedmoor. She thinks that most instances of abuse result from fits of temper or the misguided assumption that physical retribution will somehow make a mental patient behave normally. In one case of flagrant brutality against a woman patient, in 1976, Mrs. Plotnick did obtain the dismissal of a female therapy aide, because she had attacked the patient so viciously and injured her so severely. The therapy aide had punched the patient, then had dragged her down the hall by the hair from the women's dormitory to the women's bathroom, ordered the patients inside the bathroom to get out, and proceeded to work the patient over thoroughly and break her nose. By the time the aide and her bleeding victim emerged from the bathroom, enough witnesses had accumulated among patients and staff to discredit the version of the incident that the aide presented to the arbitrator. Mrs. Plotnick also succeeded in disciplining a drunk male therapy aide who attempted to commit a homosexual act with a patient in a utility closet (the patient was sober and strong and fended off his assailant), although on this occasion the aide received what was considered a light penalty — a six-month suspension — because the arbitrator found him "contrite." The aide was dismissed a year later, however, for having a bloody fight with another employee in a Creedmoor parking lot. Mrs. Plotnick recently had a male cleaner dismissed for engaging in a sexual act with a female patient. Sexual relations of any variety between staff and patients are forbidden.

⸍ ⸍ ⸍

The supposedly simpler problem of seeing to it that patients stay at the hospital — the kind that involved Sylvia Frumkin on July 7, 1978 — accounts for Creedmoor's (and Clearview's) largest category of reported incidents each year. Fifty-five of the 160 incidents recorded at Clearview in 1978 were

LWOCs or escapes. Most of the patients involved in these incidents just slipped away quietly. One pushed past a numbers man — a Creedmoor employee — who was coming inside on the daily rounds he made among the staff. Some left with a romantic liaison in mind. (There have been numerous marriages between released Creedmoor patients.) The most common reason was that the patient was simply tired of the hospital and wanted a change of scene. Few of the patients who left Creedmoor without permission in 1978 caused harm, although one man broke all the windows in his girlfriend's apartment and a woman destroyed everything in her sister's apartment. Most patients went directly home. Those who didn't usually did no more than irritate the people who live around the hospital by trespassing or urinating on their lawns, or give someone a fright by walking into a house through an unlocked front door. Theoretically, the disappearance of a patient should be discovered within a few hours, because there are six official counts daily — one at every change of shift and at mealtimes — and a number of informal counts. Counts are sometimes inaccurate, however. The staff doesn't always know who has been discharged, who has grounds privileges, and who has home leave. Occasionally, the Clearview staff first hears of a patient's departure when a relative calls to say that the patient has come home.

The failure or unwillingness of the Clearview unit's staff to fill out a Form 147 was not the only reason that most incidents of all kinds — LWOCs and escapes, medication errors, "sexual acting out," patient assaults on staff, staff abuse of patients — went unreported to higher authorities in 1978. There was another process at work within the hospital and state bureaucracy — one that might be called the disappearing-incidents syndrome. Of the 160 incidents that were written up on Form 147s in 1978 — out of the roughly 900 incidents of all types that Mrs. Plotnick estimates to have occurred in the unit — very few were written up fully. Some of the forms contained nothing but a comment by a staff member who had witnessed the incident; some had comments by that staff member and a doctor; some had been filled out by Mrs. Plotnick as well. A number of these 160 incident reports never got any further than Mrs. Plotnick's desk. Because Mrs. Plotnick is a capable administrator, she had handled incident reports by the book during her first year as chief of the Clearview unit, in 1974–75, and as a result the Clearview unit had the highest number of reported incidents in the hospital that year. Some of Mrs. Plotnick's colleagues discouraged her from exercising her administrative talent so vigorously. In the future, when she received reports of incidents that seemed minor or unlikely to have repercussions — for example, when the patient fell but wasn't seriously hurt, or escaped but came back within a few hours — she could just file these reports in the unit instead of sending them on to the Administration Building for the Incident Review Committee. If the incident should later turn into something major, she could always forward the report at that time. When Alexander Morton died after the fight on October 13, 1978, she forwarded incident reports of fights in which he had been involved on October 6 and October 10.

Of the 160 incident reports that reached her desk in 1978, Mrs. Plotnick ended up forwarding about 120 to the Administration Building. There the hospital's Incident Review Committee reviewed them and chose to forward 79 to the nearest regional office of the New York State Office of Mental Health, in Manhattan. The regional office sent these 79 incident reports — not quite half of the 160 reported to Mrs. Plotnick, and fewer than a tenth of the 900 she estimates to have occurred — on to the central office, in Albany.

Sylvia Frumkin's LWOC on July 7, 1978, was not one of the 79 incidents reported to Albany. And just as the senior hospital administrators and higher-level bureaucrats willed themselves into taking a restricted view of the reality in Creedmoor's wards by encouraging Mrs. Plotnick to restrict the number of incident reports, so those responsible for Miss Frumkin's departure on July 7 availed themselves of the paperwork process to turn it into a non-event, for which they had no responsibility.

At three-forty-five on the afternoon of July 7, Mrs. Plotnick went to the chart room to find Dr. Batra. She had him fill out a Form 147 on Miss Frumkin's disappearance, for the purpose of making sure that the record showed he had given her permission to go to Jewish services. With the same purpose in mind, she also instructed him to make a similar notation in Miss Frumkin's chart. Dr. Batra wrote on the Form 147:

> 4 P.M. — The pt. was allowed to attend the Jewish Service and later was at the Transitional Services, very upset. I called the Safety to bring pt. to the ward. She was accompanied to Bldg. N on the hall. She was not brought in the ward that she escaped.

He then wrote in the chart:

> I allowed her to go to the Jewish Services at 9:30 A.M. Later Transitional Services called me up that pt. was there very upset. I called the security officer Mr. Ragland that pt. be brought to the ward. According to him two safety officers accompanied her to Clearview Unit at the hallway. She was not brought in the ward so pt. escaped. Safety officer & father notified.

While Mrs. Plotnick accomplished her purpose by getting Dr. Batra to acknowledge that he had given Miss Frumkin permission to leave the ward, so that no one else on the team could be held responsible for having let her go without the doctor's permission, anyone from outside the unit who was ignorant of the circumstances would have no way of knowing from his notations that he bore any blame. There was no mention of Miss Frumkin's behavior, which might have indicated her mental state at the time he had let her out, and no mention of what he had allowed her to wear to Jewish services. Reading what Dr. Batra had written, a stranger might well get the impression that whatever had happened to Miss Frumkin was entirely the fault of the Safety Department.

The Creedmoor safety officers were no less adept at paperwork, or the deliberate lack of it, than Dr. Batra was. There was nothing in the safety log to show that Dr. Batra had called at midmorning with a request that the officers pick up Miss Frumkin at Transitional Services and bring her back to Clearview. Nor did the safety log say that the officers had left her in the Clearview corridor instead of taking her into the locked ward. Safety's sole log entry on Miss Frumkin for July 7 read:

> 15:30 Dr. Batra called stating that Patient Sylvia Frumkin from Building #4, Ward 043, had left on L.W.O.C.

Miss Frumkin's July 7 departure was not the first instance, or the last, in which there were disparities between Safety's version of an event and the version recorded by the staff of one of the units.

Other entries in Miss Frumkin's chart for July 7 told even more about the way Creedmoor functioned. The chart said that she had taken her oral medication in the morning. She had in fact refused it and had then been given an injection on the porch by the nurse. The chart did not record the administering of any injection to Miss Frumkin. The chart did record that she had taken her regular oral medication at one o'clock in the afternoon. She had left the ward around nine-thirty in the morning for Jewish services, and the police had brought her back at eight o'clock that night.

Mrs. Plotnick was not surprised that on July 7 Miss Frumkin had twice been credited with taking oral medication she either had not accepted or had not been present to refuse, or that the shot she had received had not been charted: Charting errors were often brought to her attention by Clearview's medical-records technician, and no amount of lecturing the staff on the importance of accurate charting seemed to change matters for very long. A few months after Miss Frumkin's LWOC, Mrs. Plotnick was shown a note written by a night-shift therapy aide. It said, "Patient slept soundly." The sound sleeper had been discharged several days earlier. In March of 1979, the medical-records technician brought her a sampling of charts. According to these charts, numerous patients had taken their medication on February 29 and February 30, 1979.

Seven

Though Miss Frumkin's LWOC did not have serious consequences for her on July 7 — she wasn't run over, she wasn't molested — she did suffer a setback after her return. On July 9, she lost a gold wedding band belonging to Barbara Herbert. Mrs. Herbert spent most of July 9 and July 10 trying to bite Miss Frumkin; she succeeded on July 11. Miss Frumkin seemed more troubled about having been bitten than about having lost Mrs. Herbert's ring, although she did ask a few other patients and staff members if she could borrow two hundred dollars from them so that she could replace the ring. She told them that Mrs. Herbert's husband had bought the gold wedding band at Tiffany's. Miss Frumkin took her 500 milligrams of Thorazine three times a day on July 9 and July 10, but she refused to take it on the mornings of the eleventh and twelfth. When she again refused her oral medication on the morning of the thirteenth, Dr. Batra wrote on the doctor's order sheet that she be given a 50-milligram injection of Thorazine three times that day — at 11:45 A.M., at 3:00 P.M., and at 6:00 P.M.

On the morning of Friday, July 14, Miss Frumkin ran to the chart room. This time, she found Stephanie Fulton there. She told Miss Fulton she wanted to go to Jewish services.

Miss Fulton felt that Miss Frumkin was still too agitated and hostile to go out alone, and said no. Miss Frumkin became even more agitated and hostile. Miss Fulton asked Miss Frumkin's social worker to call Creedmoor's rabbi and ask him to visit Miss Frumkin in the ward, in the hope that the prospect of such a visit would make her feel less deprived. It didn't. That evening, Miss Frumkin got into a fistfight with two other women in the ward. On July 15, she refused to take her medication, fought with a number of other patients, became more incoherent than she had been at any other time since her admission, and was taken to an unlocked seclusion room by a therapy aide on the night shift. She spent the night there, engaging in behavior of a particularly primitive kind, and had to be showered the next morning.

Dr. Batra had reviewed Miss Frumkin's medication again on July 14. He had ordered that from Monday to Friday she be given three 100-milligram injections of Thorazine between the hours of eight o'clock in the morning and five o'clock in the afternoon. In addition, she was to continue to receive the 500 milligrams of Thorazine orally three times a day. She took all the medicine prescribed for her — 1800 milligrams of Thorazine — on Monday, July 17. That night, she and another patient stayed up pestering the other women in the dormitory and keeping them awake until morning. On July 18, she refused the oral Thorazine. On July 19, she insisted on completely disrobing to have her blood pressure taken before accepting a Thorazine injection from a nurse on the daytime shift. A few hours later she wrestled with the licensed practical nurse on the evening shift, because she wanted to get into a seclusion room where one of her enemies was locked up. She refused her evening medication, and she tried — unsuccessfully — to get the nurse to hit her. Her behavior remained the same on July 20.

July 21 was Miss Frumkin's thirty-sixth day at Creedmoor. Not only was she not in any condition to be discharged, as almost half the people admitted to Creedmoor in 1978 were by their thirty-sixth day, but Miss Fulton didn't believe she was in any condition to go alone anywhere outside the ward. When Miss Frumkin came into the chart room that morning and once more demanded to go to Jewish services, Miss Fulton again said no. Miss Frumkin slapped Miss Fulton's face and sprinted off to the dayhall. The day was hot and humid. Neither of the two fans in the dayhall was working. Miss Frumkin seemed unaware of the weather. That morning, she was wearing a blouse, a vest, a pair of blue jeans, and a quilted jacket. She had tied another pair of blue jeans around her neck. She also wore around her neck a chain with a pop top from a soda can on it. On her feet were a pair of socks and the high-heeled gold sandals. On her head was a bandanna. Knotted into the bandanna was a spoon. "The spoon looks a little stupid, but it keeps my posture good," Miss Frumkin explained to a patient who had told her that spoons were eating utensils. She was sexually active, and pursued a number of male patients ardently — especially the profoundly retarded patient named Kevin Kiernan, who she insisted was Jesus Christ. She was sporadically nasty. She grabbed other patients' chairs and possessions, insisting that they were hers. She was also hyperactive: She danced on top of the ward's coffee tables, frequently burst into song, ran around the ward begging other patients and their visitors for money, and outtalked everyone else on the premises.

"I'm going to marry Geraldo Rivera," she told Eileen O'Reilly that day. "I think we're going to get married in Madison Square Garden, just like Sly Stone did. Mick Jagger wants to marry me. If I have Mick Jagger, I don't have to covet Geraldo Rivera. Mick Jagger is St. Nicholas and the Maharishi is Santa Claus. I want to form a gospel rock group called the Thorn Oil, but Geraldo wants me to be the music critic on *Eyewitness News,* so what can I do? Got to listen to my boyfriend. Teddy Kennedy cured me of my ugliness. I'm pregnant with the son of God. I'm going to marry David Berkowitz and get it over with. Creedmoor is the headquarters of the American Nazi Party. They're eating the patients here. Archie Bunker wants me to play his niece on his TV show. I work for Epic Records. I'm Joan of Arc. I'm Florence Nightingale. The door between the ward and the porch is the dividing line between New York and California. Divorce isn't a piece of paper, it's a feeling. Forget about Zip Codes. I need shock treatments. The body is run by electricity. My wiring is all faulty. A fly is a teen-age wasp. I'm marrying an accountant. I'm in the Pentecostal Church, but I'm considering switching my loyalty to the Charismatic Church."

A therapy aide approached Miss Frumkin. "Seclusion for two hours — Dr. Sun's orders," she said. "It ain't smart to go around hitting treatment-team leaders, now, is it?" She walked Miss Frumkin to the seclusion room and locked her in.

Dr. Sun had returned from his vacation on July 17. By July 21, he had read Miss Frumkin's chart. He was troubled by her lack of improvement on Thorazine. After observing her behavior for several days, he decided that the time had come to change her medication. Dr. Sun had had good luck with many agitated patients by prescribing an antipsychotic drug called Haldol. He figured that it would be wise to try it on Miss Frumkin, because she was obese. She was five feet four inches tall, and her weight was over 170 pounds. There are a score of antipsychotic drugs on the American market, and most of them cause patients to gain weight, but Haldol generally causes less of a weight gain. Starting on July 22, he wrote in Miss Frumkin's chart, she was to receive thirty milligrams of Haldol liquid at eight o'clock in the morning and at eight o'clock at night. She was to be given three ten-milligram injections of Haldol three times a day — at nine and eleven in the morning and at one o'clock in the afternoon — for seven straight days.

Within three days of Miss Frumkin's going on the Haldol regimen, her condition improved. She became somewhat calmer. She ran around less. She talked a little less, and what she said made a little more sense. Her clothing was less outlandish: She wore blouses and skirts, or blouses and slacks, or dresses, and plain shoes. She no longer said that she was Mary Poppins, Joan of Arc, and Florence Nightingale. She was simply Sylvia Frumkin.

On Friday, July 28, the last day of the Haldol series, Miss Frumkin went to the chart room and quietly asked Dr. Sun if she could go to Jewish services. She spoke in a pleasant tone. She was wearing a sleeveless cotton dress and a pair of brown loafers. She had taken her medicine all week uncomplainingly. She had not tangled with any of the other patients or with any members of the staff. Dr. Sun gave Miss Frumkin permission to go to Jewish services. She thanked him, walked to the Assembly Hall, and took part in the prayers. After the services, she made a halfhearted attempt to convert the rabbi to Christianity. When the rabbi told her he was comfortable with the Jewish faith, she changed the subject and said she had enjoyed the services. After eating three cheese sandwiches and two Drake's coffee cakes and drinking four cups of fruit punch, she walked back to the ward. That afternoon, the rabbi called Harriet and Irving Frumkin to say that he thought Sylvia was out of the deep sickness.

Eileen O'Reilly noticed the sudden change in Miss Frumkin and asked her how she accounted for it. "What made your mind suddenly snap back?" she asked.

"The medicine does it and prayer does it," Miss Frumkin said. "It just happens."

A psychiatrist whose specialty is psychopharmacology later reviewed Miss Frumkin's treatment and medication record. He had no trouble explaining her sudden improvement. "She was finally getting an adequate dose of medication," he said, with irritation. "Ninety milligrams of Haldol is the equivalent of forty-five hundred milligrams of Thorazine. The greatest amount of Thorazine she ever received was eighteen hundred milligrams, and that wasn't enough. There are two main ways to medicate a psychotic patient. You can start with what is called a loading dose — a high dose — and gradually decrease it. That's useful for the disturbed patient, but there are certain risks involved. For example, there is a higher incidence of side effects, including seizures, so I usually avoid loading doses except where the risk that the illness is creating for the patient is greater than the risk of the side effects. Starting low and gradually increasing the dosage is generally the preferable method. If you watch the patient carefully and find that he or she continues to act very disturbed, you should realize that you're going too slowly, and you should increase the medication faster. If this patient had been given a sufficient amount of Thorazine, Haldol, or one of the other antipsychotics much earlier, I think she would have improved much more rapidly. It's extremely unfair to patients not to medicate them aggressively, and it's extremely unfair to everyone else in the ward, who has to live with undermedicated patients, including the hospital staff that has to take care of them. One trouble is that most psychiatrists simply don't know enough about psychopharmacology. With the exception of the field of allergy, there is no field in medicine with such a range of possible doses. Each patient metabolizes these medicines differently. You have to constantly make adjustments. When I teach courses in psychopharmacology, I often find myself saying that it's like learning to drive a car. As you first learn to drive, you think you can just hold the steering wheel and the car will go straight. But you have to constantly make adjustments to keep the car on your side of the road. There's another trouble with medicating patients at hospitals like Creedmoor. The bureaucrats in Albany send down regulations that tell the doctors how much of a particular medication they're allowed to prescribe. At Creedmoor, you can't go above sixteen hundred milligrams of Thorazine without getting special permission, although at other hospitals you can raise a patient to forty-five hundred milligrams — and it's safe if you do it gradually. New York State's ceilings are arbitrary and sometimes pernicious, because they tend to restrain doctors. At Creedmoor, doctors can give up to one hundred milligrams of Haldol without getting special permission. Switching to Haldol from Thorazine is one way of getting around a perfectly arbitrary ceiling. In this case, it should have been done much sooner."

⸙ ⸙ ⸙

Once Miss Frumkin was over the six weeks of what the rabbi had called her deep sickness, she was sometimes willing to look back on certain things that had happened during that period. Her memory was selective. On July 31, she was sitting quietly in a chair, leafing through a magazine, when she was hit in the face by a patient whose condition was taking a turn for the worse as hers was taking a turn for the better. She was outraged and went over to one of the black therapy aides she had hit in June, to complain about the woman who had just hit her. When the therapy aide didn't express sufficient sympathy to suit her, Miss Frumkin said, "You should go back to Africa, where you came from."

"Sylvia, you shouldn't talk like that to any of us," the therapy aide told her. "I took care of you when you were really sick. When you cursed me out and hit me, I accepted it, because you couldn't help yourself. When you soiled yourself, we showered you and washed down the seclusion room. Now you know better than to talk like you just did."

Miss Frumkin denied to the therapy aide that she had ever hit her. Later, she said to another patient, "If I did hit her, she probably deserved it."

There were other things that had happened during those six weeks that Miss Frumkin didn't mind talking about when she was in the mood to reminisce. Just as she vividly remembered her adventures on Hillside Avenue the day Dr. Batra had let her go to Jewish services, she remembered falling in the bathroom at Transitional Services on June 16, and the subsequent trip to the emergency room of Long Island Jewish-Hillside Medical Center and from there to Clearview. She remembered the visit to the emergency room in precise detail. She remembered that when the nurse examined her she hadn't heard her say, "Stick out your tongue and say 'ah' "; she'd heard her say, "Stick out your tongue and say 'hah,' " and she remembered telling her, "That's a great idea, and it will probably win you the next Nobel Prize." One day in the fall of 1978 when Miss Frumkin was in a particularly mellow mood, she recalled how in the early-morning hours of June 16 she had believed that she was Mary Magdalene, that Paul McCartney was singing specially to her, that she was making a movie, and that Creedmoor was a police academy. She laughed and said, "I can't to this day figure out how I could have thought all those things at once."

There were also things that Miss Frumkin said she didn't remember. She said that her first two weeks back at Creedmoor were a blur. She said that she knew she had spent a lot of time in the seclusion room but didn't know why she had been put there, and she clearly didn't want to know why. She had scars from some of the bites she had received from Barbara Herbert in June and July. She showed them off in early August as if she had been an altogether innocent victim. When Eileen O'Reilly reminded her that Mrs. Herbert had bitten her on one occasion because she had lost Mrs. Herbert's wedding ring, Miss Frumkin told Miss O'Reilly that that wasn't a good enough reason to bite her — "and, anyway, the wedding band was just a two-dollar piece of junk, nothing worth getting upset over."

Miss O'Reilly was curious about all the things that Miss Frumkin had said about herself and her family before her mind snapped back. She knew that Miss Frumkin's marriages to Geraldo Rivera and Paul McCartney and John Travolta were delusions, and that writing J. R. R. Tolkien's books fell into the same category, but she wondered about some of the other statements Miss Frumkin had been making for weeks. "Tell me what I said," Miss Frumkin proposed. "It will be like playing *This Is Your Life.*"

Miss O'Reilly, who had listened to Miss Frumkin's monologues so often that she thought she could recite them herself, contradictions and all, asked Miss Frumkin first about her family. It turned out that Miss Frumkin was born in Brooklyn on May 5, 1948, and that she was the tallest person in her short family, just as she had said. She did have a sister named Joyce, who was five years and seven months older than she was, and who was a successful fashion executive. The Frumkins had moved from Brooklyn to Queens when Sylvia was four, not when she was seven or nine, and she sometimes thought that the move was the cause of her mental illness, because she had had a few nice playmates in Brooklyn. After the move to Queens, she hadn't been able to make friends with any children except those she considered losers, like her. Her grandmother had lived with the family and had died four weeks after Miss Frumkin's eighteenth birthday. Aunt Lottie had come to live with the Frumkins after the grandmother's death; in fact, Miss Frumkin's father had recently told her that Aunt Lottie had become so senile that the Frumkins had finally had to put her in a nursing home. Miss Frumkin now said that she was glad, because she hated Aunt Lottie. "I don't like most people," she told Miss O'Reilly. Miss Frumkin also had a Great-Aunt Goldie and a Great-Uncle Simon. She looked puzzled when Miss O'Reilly asked her why her Uncle Simon had thrown her into a swimming pool at the University Settlement Camp. "He didn't," she said. She thought about it for a while. "I never went to the University Settlement Camp," she said. "Joyce did. She had a counselor there named Simon. Joyce kept saying she couldn't swim. One day, after Simon had spotted her paddling along the edge of the pool when she thought he wasn't looking, he picked her up, tossed her into the pool, and told her, 'Never say can't, always say try.' Joyce was a good swimmer from then on. The story was repeated in the family whenever anyone said they couldn't do something — usually me."

"What about the cat, Sylvia?" Miss O'Reilly asked. "Did you really kill your cat?"

"We did have a cat named Gingersnap," Miss Frumkin

said. "I didn't kill it, but my mother always accused me of torturing Gingersnap by playing too hard with her. The cat lived to a ripe old age."

Miss Frumkin seemed pleased when Miss O'Reilly asked about "all those schools you went to." She told Miss O'Reilly that she had gone to the High School of Music and Art and had had to repeat the eleventh grade the following year at a private school. She looked at Miss O'Reilly in amazement when Miss O'Reilly asked her when the High School of Music and Art had become a furniture store. "I said that?" was all she would say on the subject. Miss O'Reilly recalled several names that Miss Frumkin had kept repeating — names that were unfamiliar to her, like Claude Kirchner, Bob Keeshan, and Camilla Costello, who Miss Frumkin had told her was Abbott and Costello's daughter. Miss Frumkin told Miss O'Reilly that Bob Keeshan was the name of the actor who played Captain Kangaroo and that Claude Kirchner was an actor who played the part of a ringmaster on a TV show she had watched years ago. She said that Camilla Costello was the best friend she had ever had —"and since she can't be Abbott and Costello's daughter, she must have been their niece." She told Miss O'Reilly that she couldn't believe she had said all the things that Miss O'Reilly was asking her about, but she acknowledged that she must have, because there was no other way Miss O'Reilly could have learned the name of her best friend, Camilla Costello. One of the few things she did remember saying was that the entrance to the porch was the dividing line between California and New York; she seemed enchanted by that idea. When Miss O'Reilly observed that Miss Frumkin had a marvelous memory, even if she didn't always know the dividing line between fact and fiction, Miss Frumkin said, "Yes, that's true. I've always said that I'm an idiot savant."

One day, Miss O'Reilly asked Miss Frumkin which star she most wanted to marry — Paul McCartney, Mick Jagger, Geraldo Rivera, or John Travolta. Miss Frumkin got angry when John Travolta's name was mentioned. "I'd never even consider marrying John Travolta," she said. "He's much too young for me." Then, after her anger had subsided, she said, "The others, yes. Paul McCartney, sure. I was once a real Beatles fan. And Geraldo did so much good by exposing Willowbrook. And I read somewhere that Mick Jagger and his wife split up, so maybe he's available. You know, it was fun believing some of those things I believed, and in a way I hate to give up those beliefs. I'll miss having those fantasies. There's a charm to being sick. I like to be in the twilight zone of the real world. Absolutely real is getting up every day and going to work. I once thought, when I was about to finish medical-secretarial school, before I had a breakdown on the last day of school, that I'd graduate and get a job. I was looking forward to earning my own money, to having a credit card, to being a grown woman in my own right. If you can work and earn money, you can spend money to buy Barbara Herbert a new ring. You can buy new clothes instead of wearing state clothes. And you can have fun. But if you can't have any of those things . . ." Miss Frumkin's voice trailed off, and when she started to talk again she spoke softly and in an uncharacteristically reflective tone. "When you know all those things exist for other people but not for you, sometimes it's very hard to endure the not having."

⸍ ⸍ ⸍

After her return from Jewish services on July 28, Miss Frumkin had gone directly to the chart room to see Dr. Sun, who was seated at a long table talking to a nurse. "You see, patient he came back, just like promised," Miss Frumkin said, smiling as she took advantage of this opportunity to mimic Dr. Sun's grammar and his Chinese accent. She plunked herself down in a chair across the table from Dr. Sun and asked him if she could have grounds privileges. Dr. Sun got up, went over to the chart rack, pulled out her chart, and sat down again. He quickly flipped the pages to the latest doctor's order sheet, told her she could start going out alone on the grounds for two hours a day starting Monday,

July 31, and wrote out an order to that effect. Grounds privileges were almost always first given to a patient for an hour or two a day; if, after several days, the patient didn't misuse the privileges, the hours were gradually increased. Later, passes were given allowing the patient to go home for a few hours, then for a day, then for two or three days or more. After Dr. Sun had finished writing the order, he told Miss Frumkin that her condition had improved, and that he planned to start her on lithium — the medication that psychiatrists almost always use on patients whom they have diagnosed as manic-depressives. As he spoke, Miss Frumkin looked at her chart, which was directly in front of Dr. Sun, facing him. Reading upside down is one of Miss Frumkin's talents. It has enabled her, over the years, to read many things not intended for her eyes. On this occasion, she read that she had been diagnosed as a manic-depressive when Dr. Sun had admitted her to Clearview, on June 16. "That's wrong," she told Dr. Sun firmly. "I've never been a manic-depressive. I'm a schizophrenic. I've always been a schizophrenic. Anyway, two or three other doctors have already given me lithium, after Thorazine, Stelazine, Mellaril, Prolixin, and Haldol didn't work. I like the idea of lithium — it's a natural element, found in water — but each time I was given lithium I got worse, so the doctors took me off it pretty quickly. They gave me Moban at Hillside for the first time last April. It made me feel a little high, but I was doing pretty well on it before I fell in the bathroom at Transitional. I'd like to go back on Moban."

Dr. Sun didn't contradict Miss Frumkin when she told him she was a schizophrenic. A few months later, the chief psychiatrist at Clearview and the chief psychiatrist at Creedmore also disagreed with Dr. Sun's diagnosis. Clearview's chief psychiatrist had observed Miss Frumkin on a number of occasions. He believed that she had a thought disorder rather than a mood disorder — that is, her symptoms were more characteristic of schizophrenia than of manic-depressive disorder. She was never as exhilarated as any of the patients he diagnosed as manic-depressives, and he considered her incapable of doing most of the kinds of things that manic-depressive patients were celebrated for doing — standing on the street and handing out dollar bills, going out and buying a Cadillac on an impulse, placing long-distance calls to old friends in the middle of the night. He couldn't imagine Miss Frumkin being able to drive a car, and he doubted whether she had any old friends to call. Creedmoor's chief psychiatrist, who was familiar with Miss Frumkin's case history, said that the gradual deterioration of her condition over the years was characteristic of schizophrenics, and not of manic-depressives. Dr. Sun had never read Miss Frumkin's case history, even after it came to the ward from Clearview's central files. He had a large case load at the hospital and a second job working part time at a private clinic in the Bronx. In 1979, Dr. Sun was given a brief synopsis of Miss Frumkin's case history by a colleague. "I guess my diagnosis was wrong," he said.

Dr. Sun also said that his diagnosis of Miss Frumkin had had no bearing on the medication he prescribed for her. He said that he believed he had treated her acute symptoms correctly with Thorazine and Haldol in June and July of 1978. He pointed out that he hadn't given her lithium at the end of July, when she told him that lithium hadn't been beneficial to her in the past. Dr. Sun knew that lithium was sometimes given to schizophrenics who hadn't responded well to other antipsychotic drugs, and he had read studies purporting to show that some of these patients were helped by lithium. By the same token, the antipsychotic drugs customarily given to schizophrenics were given to manic-depressives who hadn't responded well to lithium, and he had read some studies purporting to show that some of these patients were helped by the antipsychotic drugs. Many psychiatrists have learned that patients are often right about which medication has and has not helped them. It had been Dr. Sun's experience that even patients who were less articulate and less knowledgeable about drugs than Miss Frumkin were correct when they told him, "Doctor, the red pills help me and the green pills don't." Dr. Sun had never used Moban on a patient before, but he prescribed a moderate dose of it for Miss Frumkin—a hundred milligrams a day, starting on August 1. Many of the old-time doctors at Creedmoor have become cynical about the seemingly serendipitous course that events at the hospital have often taken. One of Miss Frumkin's former doctors said in 1979, "First, you turn a schizophrenic into a manic-depressive and then you fail to prescribe lithium. It just goes to show that that old proverb 'Two wrongs don't make a right' doesn't apply at Creedmoor, where two wrongs may well be required to make a right."

The specialist in psychopharmacology who had disapproved of Miss Frumkin's undermedication on Thorazine shook his head in disbelief when he learned about this change in medication. "Going from ninety milligrams of Haldol to a hundred milligrams of Moban is irrational," he said. "Ninety milligrams of Haldol is equivalent to roughly four hundred and fifty milligrams of Moban. Bureaucratic regulations at Creedmoor don't permit daily doses of Moban as high as four hundred and fifty milligrams, and the company that manufactures Moban — it's one of the newer drugs, and came on the market in 1974 — was careful to say in its advertisements that the long-term safety of four hundred milligrams a day hadn't been established. But Creedmoor does sanction up to two hundred and twenty-five milligrams of Moban a day, and the manufacturer says that that dose may be required in patients with severe symptoms. In any case, a drop to a hundred milligrams of Moban is definitely too sudden. What you want to do is gradually reduce the medication that works to a maintenance dose, which is often approximately one-third of the peak dose. What I would have done was continue the patient on Haldol and gradually reduce the dose. The Haldol hadn't given the patient any unpleasant side effects, and it seemed to be working. I believe I'd have gone on prescribing Haldol, because I believe in sticking with a winning horse."

Eight

On Monday, July 31, Miss Frumkin spent an hour on the grounds. The first thing she did after returning to the ward was to telephone her parents to say that she had enjoyed her grounds privileges and to tell them about the change in her medication. After the Frumkins had spoken to Sylvia, Mr. Frumkin called Dr. Sun and said that he and Mrs. Frumkin wanted to see him. Dr. Sun gave the Frumkins an appointment for two o'clock on August 2.

The last time Mrs. Frumkin had seen Sylvia was on Sunday, June 11 — eleven days after she arrived at Transitional Services and five days before her fall in the bathroom. Sylvia had come home that Sunday for a few of her clothes to take to her room at Transitional. (Between February 6 and May 31, when Sylvia had been hospitalized, first at Hillside and then at Creedmoor, she hadn't needed her own clothes.) In 1978, Father's Day fell on Sunday, June 18. Joyce Frumkin had had an out-of-town business trip scheduled for that weekend, so the Frumkins had celebrated Father's Day a week early, on the eleventh. Joyce Frumkin had treated her parents and her sister to dinner at one of their favorite seafood restaurants, in Hollis, Queens. In the restaurant, Joyce had noticed that Sylvia reached impulsively for a piece of bread as soon as the waiter set the bread basket on the table, and had been pleased to see that Sylvia quickly put the bread back, saying she was trying to diet. Sylvia had bolted her meal down in her usual fashion, Joyce observed, but, between mouthfuls, had been less antagonistic to her sister than usual. Joyce had driven Sylvia back to Transitional Services after dinner; on the way, the two sisters had had a civil conversation about politics; Sylvia had said she'd been reading about New York State's gubernatorial candidates and wanted to discuss them with Joyce before she voted in November. Mrs. Frumkin had spoken to Sylvia on the telephone a couple of times during the following week. Sylvia had sounded all right. On the morning of Friday, June 16, Mrs. Frumkin had telephoned Mrs. Plotnick about a matter involving Concerned Citizens for Creedmoor — a group of people, many of them relatives of patients in the hospital, who were interested in the quality of treatment provided there. Concerned Citizens had established an annual award to be given to an outstanding therapy aide at Creedmoor. Mrs. Frumkin, an active member, had been calling Mrs. Plotnick to tell her that a Clearview therapy aide had been selected to receive the Concerned Citizens' Mahata of the Year plaque for 1978. When Mrs. Plotnick's secretary buzzed her to say that Mrs. Frumkin was on the line, Mrs. Plotnick had assumed that she was calling about Sylvia's return to the unit. But after Mrs. Frumkin had greeted her cheerfully and started to talk about the mahata award, Mrs. Plotnick realized that she hadn't yet been called by a member of the staff, in accordance with hospital routine, and didn't know the bad news. Hermine Plotnick had decided that it would be best if she told Mrs. Frumkin about Sylvia's rehospitalization. When there was a pause in Mrs. Frumkin's conversation, Mrs. Plotnick had said, "I'm sorry to have to put a damper on your spirits, Mrs. Frumkin, but Sylvia has been readmitted to the ward." She had told Mrs. Frumkin briefly what had happened. Mrs. Frumkin not only had been upset to learn about the events of the morning of June 16, and about Sylvia's return to Creedmoor, but had been angry about the way she was given the news. Mrs. Frumkin was partial to people who spent as much time chatting on the telephone as she did — she rarely left her house, and the telephone was her major form of communication — and who were as outwardly warm as she was. She had no use for brisk and efficient executives. Later, she complained to a friend, "That Plotnick was very remiss not to call me sooner. She's a cold fish."

Shortly after Miss Frumkin was readmitted to Clearview, a member of the staff had called the Frumkins and advised them not to visit their daughter. It was advice that the Frumkins had often been given in the past. The Clearview therapy aides, many of whom had known Sylvia for eight years, didn't think it would do the Frumkins any good to see her when she was in an acute phase of her illness and her behavior was at its most hostile and bizarre. Harriet Frumkin had told the therapy aides of her husband's many ailments and of her own illnesses, and of Sylvia's adverse effect on Mr. Frumkin's ulcers and her arthritis. The aides also knew that the Frumkins — particularly Mrs. Frumkin — had a bad effect on Sylvia. "Those two women are allergic to each other," one mahata had said.

Irving Frumkin, a man who had never liked to take advice, had not followed the advice of the Clearview staff, despite the fact that he was sickly. He had come to see Sylvia at Creedmoor from time to time — as he had during her previous hospitalizations — even when she was at her worst. He had never complained to anyone that she hit him; indeed, he had admitted that she hit him only to those who had actually seen him being hit. A small, thin man who had looked ten or fifteen years older than his age for the last twenty years, Irving Frumkin lived uneasily with the memory that he had failed to respond to Sylvia's cries for psychiatric help when she was a teen-ager. He was determined not to repeat his mistakes of fifteen years before. Mr.

Frumkin had poor peripheral vision in both eyes and was a bad driver. He drove the family's 1974 Dart at a speed of about ten miles an hour. Joyce Frumkin, who drove a snappy red Volvo with her initials on the license plate, covered the six miles between Beechhurst and Creedmoor in fifteen minutes; it took Irving Frumkin fifty minutes to make the trip. Other drivers honked their horns when they were stuck behind him and cursed him when they were finally able to pass.

Harriet Frumkin had not visited Sylvia after being told to stay away. She had never learned how to drive a car, she didn't like to use public transportation, and she didn't like to drive with her husband at his snail's pace. She also didn't like to leave her house. She was especially comfortable at home in the summer of 1978, after Aunt Lottie had gone to a nursing home. She enjoyed having the kitchen to herself for the first time in fifteen years. From September to June she taught art to school-age children on weekday afternoons, but she took the summers off. She sent her husband to the grocery store to do the shopping; he was retired, she reminded him, and she wasn't, so he had more time to shop and to go see Sylvia.

Mrs. Frumkin had also stayed away from Creedmoor because she didn't like going to the hospital. She was active in Concerned Citizens, but she found the hospital as hellish as her daughter did. She hated to think that a daughter of hers had to spend time in such a place, and she hated even more to see her there. She also realized that the staff was right to tell her to stay away, because of the poor effect she had on Sylvia. Sylvia didn't have a good effect on her, either. On July 31, when a friend asked Harriet Frumkin if she hadn't missed seeing her daughter for all those weeks, she had answered, "To tell you the truth, it's been like a lovely vacation."

Harriet Frumkin had gone to the hospital only once during her daughter's first six weeks back at Creedmoor. After learning, during a telephone conversation with one of the aides, that when Sylvia was at large on July 7 she had had her bankbook with her, she had called Stephanie Fulton and asked her to take the bankbook away from Sylvia. Miss Fulton had succeeded in convincing Sylvia that her bankbook would be safer at home, and then had called Mrs. Frumkin and told her that she could pick it up at her convenience. On July 20, Harriet Frumkin had accompanied her husband to the hospital to get the bankbook. By then, Mrs. Frumkin had also learned that the Peruvian poncho and the pink blouse and skirt that Sylvia had been wearing on the day she was readmitted to Clearview were missing. The staff members had searched the ward, but they had not managed to find Sylvia's clothes. When Mrs. Frumkin came to Clearview, Miss Fulton gave her the bankbook and the Timex watch that Sylvia had been wearing on June 16, which had been locked up in a drawer. That day, Sylvia had been cavorting in the men's ward. Mrs. Frumkin had been so irate over the missing poncho and the missing pink outfit that she made no attempt to see her daughter. That evening, she had said over and over to a friend on the telephone, "It isn't enough that Sylvia has lost her mind. She has to lose all her clothes, too."

The Frumkins wanted to meet with Dr. Sun to ask him what he planned to do for Sylvia now that her condition had improved, and to tell him what they thought he ought to do for her now that she was once again at a turning point in her life. The Frumkins didn't see Sylvia as they walked through the women's and men's dayhalls on their way to Dr. Sun's small office. Dr. Sun offered them chairs. Mr. Frumkin began talking before he had taken a seat. He told Dr. Sun that he read all the newspaper articles he could find on mental illness and was familiar with the many drugs and medications. He also informed Dr. Sun that he worked on Saturday mornings as a volunteer at a clinic in Manhattan, helping the pharmacist dispense megavitamins. One of the doctors at the clinic was a well-known proponent of megavitamin therapy for schizophrenia, in which as much as a hundred times the recommended daily dose of ascorbic acid and such vitamins as niacinamide is given to patients. Mr. Frumkin told Dr. Sun he had nothing against the Moban that the doctor was giving Sylvia, but he wanted him to give her megavitamins, too.

Dr. Sun listened politely to Mr. Frumkin and replied that some hospitals did give megavitamins to patients, either alone or in conjunction with other drugs, but that Creedmoor was not one of them. Mr. Frumkin didn't tell Dr. Sun that Sylvia had already been given megavitamins several times in the past — when she was in a private hospital, when she was an out-patient, and at Creedmoor some years earlier — and that the megavitamins hadn't helped her. Mr. Frumkin also didn't tell Dr. Sun that other doctors had told him that the latest studies of megavitamins showed them to be ineffective in the treatment of schizophrenia. Irving Frumkin had heard only what he wanted to hear, and had tuned out the rest. He was a persistent man, and refused to believe that Sylvia's condition was incurable. He had only one wish in life: for Sylvia to get well before he died, so that he could rest in peace. He had convinced himself that a cure for Sylvia was just around the corner. If his morning paper had an article saying that dialysis was being tried on a small group of schizophrenic patients in Florida, he got excited over the idea that dialysis might be the answer for Sylvia. He hadn't read of any promising new treatment for schizophrenia in July of 1978, so he fell back on megavitamins.

Mrs. Frumkin interrupted her husband as he was proposing to Dr. Sun that Sylvia be given megavitamins. "Irving, your throat must hurt, you've been talking so much," she said. "Maybe you should have a drink of water." Harriet Frumkin no longer shared her husband's optimism that Sylvia could be cured. In the last several years, she had given up that hope. She compared her daughter's illness to a roller-coaster ride, and referred to the ride's ups and downs as Sylvia's "weller" and "sicker" phases; "weller" was an adjective she had contrived in the interests of accuracy, because she had stopped believing that her daughter would ever get "better." Mrs. Frumkin asked Dr. Sun what his treatment plans for Sylvia were, now that she was "weller." Before he could answer, she said that she hoped Sylvia would be able to return to Transitional Services soon but that she wanted him to proceed slowly, so that Sylvia would not be put under any of the pressure Mrs. Frumkin believed had caused so many of her previous setbacks. Dr. Sun said that he considered Transitional Services an excellent program, that the treatment team would meet to discuss Sylvia in a few days, and that he believed it was wise to go slow.

Mr. Frumkin abruptly got up to go. "Harriet, Dr. Sun is a very busy man," he said as his wife was in the midst of telling Dr. Sun how she had had to go to Sylvia's graduation from medical-secretarial school to get her diploma, because Sylvia had cracked up that day from the pressure. The Frumkins thanked Dr. Sun, left his office, and started to walk through the men's dayhall toward the women's dayhall, where they expected to find Sylvia. Mrs. Frumkin spotted Sylvia in the men's dayhall at the same time that Sylvia saw her. Mother and daughter greeted each other casually, as if they had seen each other only a few days earlier. It irritated Mrs. Frumkin to see how much weight Sylvia had put on in the past seven weeks and to see how sloppily she was dressed; her clothes were stained and torn. Mrs. Frumkin was also depressed to see how bad Sylvia's skin was.

The Frumkins had a specific reason for visiting Sylvia that day: to discuss a financial matter. They suggested to her that they sit down at an empty table in the men's dayhall to conduct their business. In 1973, after Irving Frumkin had started to draw Social Security, Sylvia Frumkin began to receive a monthly Social Security Administration disability check on her father's Social Security account. Miss Frumkin had become eligible for a monthly S.S.A. payment because she was the dependent of a retired worker who was covered by Social Security, because she was unmarried, and because she had been severely disabled before reaching the age of twenty-two. From 1973 on, she was entitled to receive the S.S.A. checks, which increased from time to time with the cost of living, whether she was in or out of a hospital. At the beginning of 1978, her monthly check was $149.

When Miss Frumkin was out of the hospital and living in the community, as she had been deemed to be doing whenever she resided at Transitional Services, she was also entitled to receive a monthly Supplemental Security Income check, which was paid for in part by the federal government and in part by New York State, and issued by the federal government. At the beginning of 1978, Miss Frumkin's monthly S.S.I. and S.S.A. checks totaled $424.70. In January, which was to be her last full month in the community that year, Transitional Services deducted $350 from her checks to cover its monthly fee for room, board, and services. Transitional Services turned over the balance — $74.70 — to her to spend on her personal needs.

It sometimes takes a while for S.S.I. checks to stop coming once a person is no longer living in the community and is thus no longer entitled to receive them. Miss Frumkin's S.S.I. checks came to Transitional Services for a few months after her return to Creedmoor on June 16. On August 1, she had gone to Transitional Services, at her parents' behest, to collect the S.S.I. checks and the S.S.A. checks that had arrived and had been held there for her during the six weeks she was confined to the ward. Mr. and Mrs. Frumkin came to Creedmoor on August 2 for the express purpose of having their daughter sign the S.S.I. checks and the S.S.A. checks, which were made out in her name, so that Mr. Frumkin could put them in the bank.

Mental patients and husbands and wives of mental patients are legally liable for paying the costs of hospitalization, or for as much of it as they can afford. Parents and children of patients are not legally liable for the costs of their care. The Office of Mental Health's Bureau of Patient Resources, an agency with the twofold purpose of recovering reimbursement and protecting patients' assets, has offices at many large state hospitals like Creedmoor, where a number of Patient Resources agents investigate the financial situation of patients and their legally liable relatives. In June of 1978, the cost of caring for a patient in a geographical unit at Creedmoor was calculated at $65.20 a day, or $23,798 a year. (By 1981, the cost had increased to $115.70 a day, or $42,230.50 a year.) Few husbands, wives, or patients could pay much of this sum from their own assets, but a certain percentage of them made partial contributions. Miss Frumkin's monthly check for $149, less $28.50, which she was legally entitled to be given as spending money, was considered by Patient Resources to be the sum she could afford to contribute to the cost of her hospitalization.

When people enter mental hospitals, a question arises concerning their ability to handle their own checks. After their admission, if the Social Security Administration determines that they are incapable of handling their own funds, someone else — usually a relative or a friend, but sometimes the director of the hospital — becomes the "representative payee," and the checks are made out to that person. Most of the relatives and friends who were representative payees for patients at Creedmoor in 1978 turned the S.S.A. checks over to the Office of Mental Health, in Albany. Irving Frumkin was one of the few exceptions. He had refused since 1974 to turn his daughter's S.S.A. checks over to the state when she was hospitalized. In early 1974, when Sylvia Frumkin was a patient at Creedmoor, Mr. Frumkin had battled with an inexperienced Patient Resources agent. He had talked the agent into letting him keep all of his daughter's monthly S.S.A. check except twenty dollars, which he agreed to send to the state. Miss Frumkin had been discharged from Creedmoor in the spring of 1974. When she was readmitted to the hospital in February of 1976, the computer had resumed billing Mr. Frumkin at the twenty-dollar-a-month rate. Sometimes he had paid the twenty dollars, sometimes he hadn't.

In late 1976, an experienced agent had reviewed the case.

She had found the account in arrears and had also decided that the twenty-dollar-a-month rate was insufficient. The agent had wanted the hospital director to become the representative payee. Meetings with the Frumkins, Sylvia, and her social worker had been held in late 1976 and early 1977. At these meetings, Mr. Frumkin had insisted that he was spending much more than $28.50 a month on Sylvia for things like new clothes — a fact disputed by the ward staff and also by his daughter. Miss Frumkin had requested that the hospital director be made representative payee, so that she would receive the $28.50 a month instead of the dollar or two her father, whom she had described at one meeting as "miserly," doled out. The staff had agreed that it would be therapeutic for Miss Frumkin to be less financially dependent on her father. In January of 1977, Mrs. Frumkin had said that she and her husband would tentatively let the director become the representative payee; several weeks later, Mr. Frumkin had called to say that he had changed his mind. The Frumkins had reached a compromise with Patient Resources in early 1977. Mr. Frumkin would remain the representative payee, but he would send the state seventy dollars a month from Sylvia's S.S.A. check instead of twenty, and he would give Sylvia the balance of the check — seventy-nine dollars — as spending money. Despite the agreement, the Frumkins had rarely made any payments to the state. Mr. Frumkin had preferred to keep the S.S.A. checks and to give his daughter a small monthly allowance. By the summer of 1978, Mr. Frumkin was no longer the representative payee; the checks were being made out directly to his daughter.

On August 2, 1978, Mr. Frumkin wanted Sylvia to sign the green S.S.A. checks and the gold S.S.I. checks she had fetched from Transitional Services the previous day. Now that she had been given grounds privileges, which Mr. Frumkin knew would soon increase, she would want money to spend. The first thing he did when he sat down at the table in the men's dayhall with his wife and daughter was to negotiate Sylvia's allowance. They settled amicably on nine dollars a week. That was her first incentive to sign the checks and give them to her father. There was a second incentive. Irving Frumkin liked to play a game that both his daughters called "musical banks." Whenever a bank advertised gifts for people who deposited a certain sum of money and agreed to keep the money there for a minimum period of time, Mr. Frumkin opened a new bank account. Harriet and Irving Frumkin's kitchen and Joyce Frumkin's kitchen contained many small appliances from banks all over New York City. Mr. Frumkin withdrew the money the day the minimum period of time was up, and deposited it in another bank then offering gifts to new depositors. On August 2, Mr. Frumkin wanted to use his daughter's S.S.A. and S.S.I. checks to open a fourteen-month bank account in his name for a thousand dollars at a bank that was proffering gifts that week. Mr. Frumkin had once told Sylvia that she couldn't have more than several hundred dollars in the bank in her own name, because the state or the federal government might one day take her money away from her, so he would open accounts "in trust" for her. (Sylvia had once gone through her parents' house while they were out, and had turned the rooms upside down looking for the bankbooks, but hadn't been able to find them. They were kept in a safe-deposit box.) Mr. Frumkin wanted the money in his name not simply to keep it from the state and the federal government — Miss Frumkin was legally entitled to have fifteen hundred dollars in assets without losing her eligibility for such programs as S.S.I. — but because his daughter was a spendthrift. He knew that if her condition improved, soon she would ask for the money and would squander it. If he had the thousand dollars tied up for fourteen months, he could tell her when she asked for it that he couldn't withdraw it. Mr. Frumkin now told Sylvia that she could choose the gift that the bank was offering new depositors — the second incentive to sign.

Mr. Frumkin had brought to the hospital a full-page bank advertisement he had cut out of a newspaper, which showed all the gifts that a bank in Manhattan was offering to those who opened accounts of two hundred and fifty, five hundred, a thousand, and five thousand dollars. While Sylvia was looking over the ad, the Frumkins were pestered by patients. A steady stream of men and women approached their table and begged for cigarettes or for quarters for vending machines in the central corridor. The three Frumkins decided to go outside. Mrs. Frumkin asked a therapy aide to let them out of the ward. They walked to their car and spread the newspaper ad out on top of the trunk for Sylvia to study.

She quickly eliminated some of the gifts in the thousand-dollar category. She didn't want a smoke-and-fire detector, a tool set, a knife set, or a carpet sweeper; her own safety had never been of concern to her, and she was clumsy with tools and knives, didn't like cleaning, and was bored by utilitarian objects. The first gift that appealed to her was an eight-digit calculator. "I could use that to tally my calories and to do my budget," she told her parents.

"What do you need a calculator for?" Mrs. Frumkin asked. "You have one at home."

"I'm at Creedmoor, I'm not at home," Sylvia said.

"It will get stolen," her mother said.

Miss Frumkin looked momentarily frustrated, but soon she noticed a digital alarm clock among the thousand-dollar-account gifts. "That would be good for waking myself up when I'm back at Transitional," she said.

"You're not at Transitional, you're on the ward," her mother said. "It would get stolen on the ward."

"You could keep it for me until I return to Transitional," Sylvia countered.

"You don't need an alarm clock," Mrs. Frumkin said. "They wake you up at Transitional. The trouble is, you don't get out of bed when they tell you to get out of bed."

Sylvia sighed. Then she spotted a hair dryer and said that that was what she wanted.

"You already have a hair dryer at home," her mother told her.

"But this one looks nicer than the one I have at home," Sylvia said.

"The one at home is good enough," Mrs. Frumkin said.

Similar exchanges followed about a tote bag ("Sylvia, you already have plenty of bags") and a portable radio ("You broke the last ten portable radios you had"). In exasperation, Sylvia turned to her mother and said, "I thought you told me I could choose."

After another quarter hour of bickering, a selection was made. Sylvia's gift would be a high-intensity lamp. She said she would keep it at home for the time being and use it in her room at Transitional Services after her return there. Sylvia later gave the lamp to her mother. In October of 1979, when her father withdrew the thousand dollars (plus six and a half percent interest) from the bank in Manhattan, Sylvia had apparently forgotten about the account and didn't ask about it. In January of 1980, when Miss Frumkin had occasion to reapply for S.S.I., she was told by an official from her local Social Security office that he had discovered that S.S.I. had overpaid her approximately seven hundred dollars after her return to Creedmoor from Transitional Services in 1978, and that she would be ineligible for S.S.I. until that amount was returned. Miss Frumkin told the official that she had given the checks to her father. Mr. Frumkin told the official that Sylvia had spent the money.

On August 2, 1978, the gift having been selected and the checks having been signed, the Frumkins drove Sylvia from the parking area near Clearview to the Transitional Services building in which she had lived until her fall in the bathroom on June 16. Miss Frumkin had left some clothes there. When the Frumkins went inside to look for them, no one seemed to know where they were. "It's not bad enough that my daughter has to lose her mind, she has to lose her clothes, too," Mrs. Frumkin said again — in front of Sylvia this time. Later, the clothes were found in a suitcase on the floor of the closet in the room that Sylvia had occupied.

Nine

In 1978, almost two-thirds of the patients who were discharged from the Clearview unit returned to their own homes. Among the many who went home was Barbara Herbert, who "snapped to" one day in August even more precipitately than Sylvia Frumkin had. Mrs. Herbert suddenly stopped biting and hitting, and became quiet and friendly; she went home on several weekend visits with her husband, and returned to live with him in early September.

One thing that Harriet, Irving, and Sylvia Frumkin and a social worker at Clearview, who was trying to help Miss Frumkin formulate some realistic plans for the future, agreed on was that it would not be in Sylvia's best interests or in her parents' best interests for her to return home. They all hoped that she could go back to Transitional Services to live. One day in early August, the Clearview social worker spoke to a counselor at Transitional Services about the possibility of Miss Frumkin's returning there in a few weeks. The counselor called back to say that she and the rest of the Transitional Services team thought that to go directly from two months of confinement in a locked ward to Transitional would be too drastic a step for Miss Frumkin to take. The counselor said that the team would be willing to consider screening Miss Frumkin for readmission to Transitional Services from the ward only after she had done well in a "program" for a month. The first thing that the social worker had to do for Miss Frumkin was to help her decide on a program.

Among the programs available on the grounds of Creedmoor in August of 1978 were adult-education courses in a variety of subjects, at a variety of levels, from grade school to high school; several "sheltered workshops"; and several day treatment centers. Miss Frumkin had never taken an adult-education course at Creedmoor; as a graduate of a private high school, with an academic diploma, she considered herself too advanced for any of the classes offered. She had, however, been a client at several of Creedmoor's sheltered workshops. She had spent a short time in early 1974 at the clerical-skills sheltered workshop, commonly referred to as the typing workshop. In 1976 and 1977, she had spent a number of months at a sheltered workshop whose clients were assigned such benchwork-assembly tasks as packaging individual sets of cutlery, napkins, and condiments for the use of airline passengers, fastening buttons to the cards on which they were to be sold, and boxing shower-curtain hooks. And she attended the Clearview Day Center for several months in 1977.

Miss Frumkin hadn't enjoyed putting plastic forks, knives, and spoons, paper napkins, packages of sugar, and tiny salt and pepper shakers into cellophane bags in the benchwork-assembly sheltered workshop. She found such tasks tiresome. Working in a factory was not one of her goals, she told the social worker when they met on August 4, 1978. She had liked her brief exposure to the typing workshop, and wanted to return there. The last job she had ever held in the outside world was working Saturdays as a receptionist in the office of the Frumkins' internist, from October 1971 to July of 1972, while she was going to medical-secretarial school during the week. She thought she might someday want to work as a receptionist again, and said that the typing workshop was the program of her choice. The social worker told her she wasn't yet ready for the typing workshop; she would first have to try a program that was less pressured. If she did well at it she could then apply to the typing workshop. Miss Frumkin hadn't cared for the Day Center when she went there in 1977 — she had found it rather like a nursery school — but she wanted to return to Transitional Services, and to be given that opportunity she needed to be in a program for a month, and so, as she told the social worker, she would go to the Clearview Day Center. It was the least of the available evils, she said.

The Clearview Day Center was a pleasant four-bedroom red brick house that had once been the home of one of Creedmoor's assistant directors; it was a five-minute walk from Building N/4. In August of 1978, most of its twenty clients were Clearview out-patients who had been discharged to their homes. The majority were middle-aged or older women who lived either with relatives or on their own with the help of some sort of subsidy. Their relatives often said that the Day Center gave them a reason to get up in the morning. Without it, the relatives said, they were afraid the clients would stay in the house all day — if not actually in bed, as some did on weekends. The Clearview Day Center had a full-time staff of five — the coordinator, two therapy aides, a recreational therapist, and an occupational-therapy assistant. The Day Center program was not rigorous. The days tended to start late and end early.

On Monday, August 14, Miss Frumkin made out her schedule with a therapy aide at the Day Center. She was to be there full time on Mondays, Tuesdays, and Thursdays, and to go there on Fridays after Jewish services and on Wednesday mornings. (By mid-August, Dr. Sun was allowing Miss Frumkin to spend two afternoons a week — Wednesdays and Sundays — with her parents.) According to her Day Center schedule, which changed slightly from week to week, she would participate in exercises for fifteen minutes every morning; in a weekly fifteen-minute client-government meeting, at which the clients discussed such matters as how much to charge for coffee each morning; in an hour-long therapeutic-community meeting held every Monday morning and attended by the staff and all the clients, at which the Day Center's current and future activities and any problems that the clients felt like bringing up were discussed; and in a weekly hour-long primary group, in which a staff member met with a smaller number of Day Center clients — usually six or seven — to discuss any personal or Day Center problems they might have. The rest of Miss Frumkin's schedule included an hour or so each week of music, drama, poetry, current events, arts and crafts, and grooming; an hour and a half of dusting, vacuuming, and washing dishes; and two hours a week of recreation, which sometimes meant bowling or swimming in the Rehabilitation Building and sometimes, in nice weather, walking in Alley Pond Park, a public park near Creedmoor frequented by drug dealers.

Miss Frumkin wasted no time before displaying her boredom with the Day Center, especially when her schedule required her to participate in an activity that wasn't to her liking. One morning in August, Miss Frumkin and five other women straggled into the master bedroom of the former assistant director's house, where the grooming class was held. The mahata in charge had put out an assortment of nail polishes and cosmetics. An elderly woman said she had filed the nails on her left hand at home but was so right-handed that she couldn't do the nails on her right hand. The woman was appreciative when the mahata filed the nails on her right hand. Another woman seemed content to apply mascara, a third to take a nap, and a fourth to wait her turn to have her nails clipped by the mahata. Miss Frumkin sat in the room looking unhappy. To make sure that her unhappiness did not go unobserved, she sighed loudly. When the mahata didn't give her the satisfaction of asking what was bothering her, she said without being asked that the grooming class was a complete waste of her time. She told the mahata and the other women in the room that she had very precise ideas about makeup. She said that she loved makeup and that she spent a good part of her allowance on moisturizers, bases, lipsticks, lip glosses, and eye makeup. When Miss Frumkin used her makeup in moderation, it covered up her blemished skin and improved her appearance. She usually came to the Day Center wearing too much makeup; her makeup was often smeared, as it was in grooming class that morning. "I use very modest makeup," she said, looking disdainfully at the bottles of pink, orange, and red nail polish that the mahata had set out. "I like colorless nail polish," she went on, holding out her hands. Those who looked at her nails saw ten badly bitten nails and ragged cuticles. Though Miss Frumkin made it obvious that she felt superior to the other clients at the Day Center, and took pleasure in putting them down whenever she could, they rarely retaliated. No one criticized her nails. "What's there for me to do?" she asked, yawning without covering her mouth.

The mahata knew how to please her and chose to do so then. "Why don't you tell the others how fast nails and hair grow?" she suggested to Miss Frumkin.

"My nails grow a tenth of an inch a week and hair grows at the rate of half an inch a month," she said happily, in a singsong voice. "I wish the nails on my hands were as hard as the nails on my feet."

⁒ ⁒ ⁒

On Sunday August 13 — the first day that Dr. Sun allowed Miss Frumkin to go home on a three-hour pass — she returned to Creedmoor saying she had had a very nice time. She had looked through the clothes in her closet; she had taken a shower, washed her hair, and enjoyed blowing it dry with her hair dryer; she had had a good Chinese dinner, her mother's usual combination of canned chow mein, canned bean sprouts, and leftover meat, served with wonton soup from a Chinese takeout in the neighborhood. Before long, when the novelty of the first couple of Wednesday and Sunday outings and visits home had worn off, and when it seemed to Miss Frumkin that her parents were less eager to please her and instead seemed bent on frustrating her, she told the staff of the Day Center that her "afternoons off" from Creedmoor were "not so good."

One Wednesday afternoon in August, her father picked her up at Clearview. He had agreed to take her to see the movie *Heaven Can Wait* and to take her shopping for a pair of sandals. Her mother had refused to join them, even though she was free to since it would be another week or so before she started giving art lessons again. Harriet Frumkin said that the movie sounded silly. *Heaven Can Wait* was being shown at a number of theaters in Queens, including two in Flushing. Mr. Frumkin drove from Creedmoor to Flushing. There were no parking spaces available near the theater. Sylvia suggested that they drive a few miles to another theater where the movie was playing — one in a neighborhood where parking was less of a problem. Her father said he was sorry but it was too late to go to another theater. He found a parking space near Main Street and took Sylvia to a number of shoe stores. She was tired of wearing state shoes, and her parents had agreed to buy her a pair of sandals on sale. The summer sandal sales had ended in all the shoe stores. The new fall shoes and boots were on display. Sylvia said she would wait until spring to buy sandals, and settled for going to a Woolworth's, where she bought an eyebrow pencil. She had hoped to go to a fast-food steak restaurant, but her father said he had some discount coupons that were valid for twelve pieces of chicken at Kentucky Fried Chicken, so they went to Kentucky Fried Chicken, bought the chicken, and drove to the Frumkins' house to eat it. The following day, there was enough chicken left over for Mr. and Mrs. Frumkin's dinner.

In mid-August, Miss Frumkin needed a haircut. She tried

to telephone Jason, her hairdresser, whom she had last seen in early June, and learned from the receptionist at the beauty parlor in Flushing where he had worked then that he had moved on to another beauty parlor, in Huntington, Long Island, about thirty miles away. Miss Frumkin called the beauty shop in Huntington and made an appointment with Jason. She had spent $10.40 of her own money for her haircut in June, while she was living at Transitional Services. When Harriet Frumkin learned that it would cost $10.40 for Jason to cut Sylvia's hair in Huntington, she told Sylvia to cancel her appointment. Mrs. Frumkin made an appointment for her at a beauty shop in Flushing, where the price of a haircut was $4.50. Her father drove her there on another Wednesday afternoon in late August. Perhaps because Sylvia looked so unhappy, or because she kept telling Sharon, the hairdresser, that Jason was the only person in the world who knew how to cut her hair, Sharon was less friendly to her than Jason had been. Sylvia complained that Sharon was careless, too. Jason had brushed the hair off Sylvia's neck and shoulders and had dusted her off with powder after he finished cutting her hair. Sharon neither brushed nor powdered her, and Sylvia left the shop feeling itchy. She also didn't like the way her haircut looked. It was too short, she thought, and no one complimented her on it. She resolved to return to Jason as soon as the haircut grew out.

In early September, Dr. Sun gave Miss Frumkin permission to spend weekends at home. Her father usually picked her up at Creedmoor on Saturday morning and drove her back to the hospital on Sunday evening or Monday morning. Sunday, September 17, was another disappointing day for Miss Frumkin. She had made arrangements to meet a young woman named Joan Bettelheim in Flushing at one o'clock. A few years earlier, Miss Bettelheim, who had often been in and out of Creedmoor, had gone to bed with a man she had met on the street. She had become pregnant and had given her child up for adoption. When she was out of the hospital, as she was in September of 1978, she lived with her father and her older sister. There was an all-day street fair in Flushing on the seventeenth. Mr. Frumkin dropped Sylvia off in Flushing promptly at one o'clock; he was to pick her up at four o'clock. Miss Frumkin had $3.00 in her purse. She waited for Miss Bettelheim for an hour. At two o'clock, she realized that she had been stood up by Miss Bettelheim — not for the first time. By then, she had spent $2.90 on food. She called home with her last dime. Her mother answered the telephone. When Sylvia told her what had happened, Harriet Frumkin told her that her father was out shopping. He would come and get her as soon as he could after he returned. Sylvia had to wait an hour and a half for him. As soon as she got home, she telephoned Miss Bettelheim to ask what had happened. Miss Bettelheim said she had changed her mind about going to the fair with Miss Frumkin. She didn't make any excuses for not having called beforehand to tell Miss Frumkin that she had changed her mind. Miss Frumkin later recounted her side of the telephone conversation to a woman at the Day Center. "I was very nice to her," she said. "I said I'd go out with her again, but the next time she'd have to come to my house to meet me, or, better yet, I'd go to her house to meet her."

Miss Frumkin often sought to convey the impression that she philosophically accepted such disappointments as broken dates, cheap haircuts, movies she couldn't see when she wanted to see them, and sandals she couldn't buy when she wanted to buy them, but by mid-September a number of people at Creedmoor had noticed that she was displaying increasing signs of tension, even when she didn't express her frustration verbally. She bit her cuticles until they bled. She ate incessantly. In mid-September, Mrs. Plotnick thought she also noticed that Miss Frumkin was smacking her lips, rolling her tongue around in her mouth, and touching her lower lip with her tongue until she made her lip sore — symptoms of tardive dyskinesia, a side effect that some patients develop from prolonged use of antipsychotic drugs. Mrs. Plotnick knew that while some psychiatrists considered tardive dyskinesia irreversible, others believed that it often was reversible and that it was certainly arrestable, especially if it was caught in an early stage and the patient was taken off antipsychotic medication or given a much lower dose. She sought out Dr. Sun and asked him to examine Miss Frumkin. Dr. Sun did. He said he believed that Miss Frumkin's tongue and lip movements were merely mannerisms.

Although Miss Frumkin tended to be indolent at home — she didn't want to clean her room, she didn't want to wash her clothes, she didn't want to get out of bed some days — she kept after her social worker in the ward with great persistence, having learned from her parents that the squeaky wheel gets the grease. She told the social worker so often that she hated the Day Center and wanted to go to the typing workshop that the social worker arranged for her to be screened by Marilyn Gruen, the coordinator of the workshop, on September 12. In Mrs. Gruen's estimation, Miss Frumkin's typing was adequate — all the people admitted to the typing workshop had to have a basic knowledge of touch-typing — but Mrs. Gruen thought that Miss Frumkin was too restless to spend a whole day at the typing workshop. She agreed to accept Miss Frumkin in the typing workshop part time, starting on Monday, September 18. In mid-September, Miss Frumkin also reminded the social worker in the ward that she had been promised she would be considered for Transitional Services after a month in a program. She had been at the Day Center for a month. The Clearview social worker called the counselor at Transitional Services and arranged for Miss Frumkin to be screened on September 28. After the screening, Miss Frumkin didn't think that it had gone well, and told the staff at the Day Center that she was afraid she had not been accepted. In the meantime, however, she was glad to be back at the typing workshop part time, and frequently told the Day Center staff that the only thing she wanted was to leave their nursery school and go to the typing workshop full time. On Sunday, September 17, while she was waiting in vain for Miss Bettelheim to show up in Flushing, she had felt glad to be starting in the typing workshop the following morning. She hadn't done well there during the brief trial period in April of 1974, and she was thankful that she was being given another chance. One reason she was eager to go to the workshop was that her mother got upset with her when she spent so much of her time at home lolling around the house. Her mother kept asking her why she was so lazy on Saturday and Sunday when "you haven't done anything all week at Creedmoor." Miss Frumkin had said to herself that on the following weekend when her mother accused her of doing nothing all week at Creedmoor, as she was sure to do, she could tell her, "I don't do nothing all week. I type."

Ten

There were twenty-seven people on the typing-workshop rolls on Monday, September 18. About half of them were out-patients. The other half were from the geographical units and from Creedmoor's forensic unit. The typing workshop's hours were from nine to eleven in the morning, with a twenty-minute coffee break at ten o'clock, and from one-thirty to three-thirty in the afternoon, with a twenty-minute coffee break at two-thirty. The typing workshop provided some of its clients with a pleasant place to go each day, just as the Day Center did, and, in addition, it gave them a chance to earn some money. Clients in the typing workshop, like those in the benchwork-assembly sheltered workshops, were paid on the basis of the 1978 federal minimum wage of $2.65 an hour. A study had been done to determine how long it took an average worker on the outside to do a thousand envelopes. The study had yielded a unit price of $28.05 per thousand envelopes. In 1978, Mrs. Gruen had some typists who could turn out a thousand envelopes a week and some who could turn out a hundred. Thus, in theory, her fastest typists could have earned $28.05 apiece each week; in practice, they rarely did, because there was usually a shortage of clerical work. "People in the community don't trust mental patients," Miss Frumkin said during a coffee break one day when the typing workshop was out of envelopes. "Contractors probably don't give us their work, because we're mental patients, so they don't think we can do a decent job." Although Mrs. Gruen and Francesa Wilcox, the assistant coordinator of the typing workshop, checked each envelope before it left their premises to make sure that it was error-free, they agreed with Miss Frumkin's appraisal of the demoralizing shortage of work. In 1978, several out-patients had been coming to the typing workshop for two or three years; one had been there for five years. Some of these out-patients credited the typing workshop with keeping them out of the hospital. Most of them knew they wouldn't be able to stand the hours and the pressures of the marketplace, but they felt comfortable in a sheltered-workshop setting. No specific minimum speed was required for people to be admitted to the typing workshop, and the clients' speeds varied greatly. Mrs. Gruen stressed accuracy rather than speed. In September of 1978, Miss Frumkin typed at a rate of thirty words a minute and made about fifteen errors a minute. Clients who typed erratically, as she did, had to practice their skills before they were permitted to type envelopes.

Only fourteen of the workshop's twenty-seven clients arrived on time on September 18 and punched in on the time clock near the door. A fifteenth came in forty-five minutes late. Mrs. Gruen and Mrs. Wilcox usually telephoned the wards of the typing workshop's missing in-patient clients. The calls were rarely fruitful. Ward extensions were often busy. (Creedmoor had too few telephones.) The therapy aides who answered the ward phones sometimes said they didn't know where Mrs. Gruen's clients were and sometimes said they didn't know who they were. The patients who were reached often said that they didn't feel like coming to the typing workshop that day, or that they were scheduled to go for X rays or to the dermatology clinic. Occasionally, Mrs. Gruen, a forceful woman, prevailed upon a recalcitrant patient to come to the typing workshop. One morning, she called a ward and reached a patient who said she had a bad cold. "You sound fine," Mrs. Gruen told her. "You've just overslept. Get yourself over here right away and bring your friend Doris with you." Both women showed up at the typing workshop in fifteen minutes. Out-patients were not called unless Mrs. Gruen had reason to be worried about them.

Miss Frumkin would have liked to start typing envelopes for money on September 18, but she accepted graciously the news that she wasn't yet ready to do envelopes. Mrs. Gruen gave her a typing book and assigned her a particular exercise to type. Miss Frumkin sat down at a free electric typewriter and raced through the exercise, making many mistakes as she typed. She ran from her desk in the middle of the room up to Mrs. Gruen's desk at the front of the room to show her the exercise. The first time she presented Mrs. Gruen with the mistake-riddled exercise, Mrs. Gruen told her to slow down and retype it with fewer errors. She was told the same thing when she ran up the second time, and the third, fourth, and fifth times. Having to retype didn't seem to bother Miss Frumkin. She was completely absorbed by typing. Since June, nothing else, in or out of the hospital, had so engaged her concentration.

If a person who had never been in a psychiatric hospital were blindfolded, escorted into the typing workshop at Creedmoor, and relieved of the blindfold, he would never mistake Creedmoor's workshop for a brushup typing class at a community college or a local Y. Most days, about a third of the clients who showed up worked quietly and diligently; they could pass for Y students. Something about the others would indicate that they had known trouble. The aftereffects of mental illness were often as visible as scars or limps left by physical injuries. One morning in October of 1978, while Miss Frumkin walked back and forth from her desk to show Mrs. Gruen or Mrs. Wilcox each exercise she pulled out of her typewriter, always speaking too quickly and in a slightly breathless way, another young woman spent the morning strutting back and forth from her typewriter to the ladies' room down the hall. No matter how often she was told to sit down and type, she rose again to walk to the ladies' room. Another woman suddenly burst into tears. Two women fell asleep at their typewriters. A woman read a paperback book on her lap. Another woman slumped in her chair and stared into space. When Mrs. Gruen told her clients, in her best no-nonsense manner, to stop crying, to wake up, or to stop reading, the clients failed to respond to her edicts. The woman who was crying couldn't stop crying. The reader and the two awakened sleepers said, "I don't feel like typing," "I don't feel well today," and "Leave me alone." Even some of those who were typing on that October morning wouldn't have struck a visiting stranger as students at a community college. Some wore perpetually dour expressions. Some appeared withdrawn, their eyes glazed. Some showed the Parkinsonian-like effects of antipsychotic medication, and some showed symptoms of tardive dyskinesia.

Miss Frumkin's eagerness to type envelopes exceeded her typing skill. In October, she continued to make too many mistakes on the exercises to advance to envelopes, but her enthusiasm for typing and her ability to accept criticism, so limited everywhere else, persisted. She typed and retyped, with uncustomary patience, the lines that were intended to help her master certain sequences of letters: "fell ill, real life, a dark red dress, like a real lake, if all jars are full, ill kill, a faded leaf, field lilies, a skillful lad, leads a dull life, a fair deal." Mrs. Gruen and Mrs. Wilcox kept telling her to slow down and relax. Every week, a short speed test was given in the workshop. In October, Miss Frumkin was allowed to take only one test. She typed at a rate of thirty words a minute and made fifteen errors a minute, just as she had in September. The workshop was Miss Frumkin's refuge. She always came to typing early or on time. She seemed particularly eager to get to typing after her weekends at home.

⸝ ⸝ ⸝

If two days at home were too much of a strain for Miss Frumkin and her parents — and they were — three-day and four-day weekends were worse. In 1978, the Jewish New Year fell on Monday, October 2, and Tuesday, October 3. Miss Frumkin went home on Saturday, September 30, and was to return to Creedmoor on Tuesday. Saturday went fairly well, because Miss Frumkin made an effort to please her mother — she cleaned her room, she did her laundry, she ate moderately. On Sunday, she stayed in bed until two o'clock, got up and ate everything she could find in the refrigerator, and then lay around. She was in her nightgown watching television when Joyce Frumkin arrived to spend the night. Sunday evening Sylvia kept the family waiting to go to temple while she put on her makeup and tried on a dozen different outfits before deciding what to wear. Joyce had come home in a good mood. She had just been promoted by the department store for which she worked, but she was careful to say nothing about her new title or her raise in salary, for fear of making Sylvia jealous. There had been many times in her life when she wished she had a sister with whom she could share her joys and sorrows. On Sunday, after temple services, Sylvia refused to help Joyce set the table, bit her lip while waiting to be served, overate, got up from the table in the middle of dinner without excusing herself, and went to her room to watch television. On Monday, while Sylvia went to temple with her father, Joyce and Harriet Frumkin prepared dinner — matzo-ball soup, gefilte fish, brisket of beef, green beans, and boiled potatoes. They had bought challah and pastries from a neighborhood bakery. Sylvia had finished her first and second plates of food and was about to start on her third before her parents and her sister had finished their first helpings. On Sunday, Joyce had restrained herself, and hadn't criticized anything Sylvia said or did; she hadn't seen her sister in more than two and a half months, and she reminded herself that Sylvia was a person to whom life had dealt a bad hand. By Monday, however, she could no longer watch in silence as Sylvia noisily slurped her soup, dipped the challah in the brisket gravy, got spots all over herself and the tablecloth, and talked with her mouth full. When Joyce criticized Sylvia's table manners and said "Slow down," Sylvia threatened to throw a plate at her. "If you weren't my sister, I'd have nothing to do with you," Joyce said.

As the dinner progressed, Mrs. Frumkin said that no one who didn't have a mentally ill child could possibly imagine what it was like. She observed that she had recently seen a couple named Isadore and Gertie Finkel, the parents of a young woman named Sonya who had often been a patient at Creedmoor. The Frumkins and the Finkels had met when their daughters were in the same ward. Sonya Finkel had tried to commit suicide several times. Her last attempt, a year earlier, had been successful: She had jumped down on the subway tracks and had been run over by a train. Her father, who had a heart condition, was retired. Her parents had wanted to move from Queens to Arizona for many years, but felt they couldn't go there as long as Sonya was in and out of Creedmoor. "After Sonya died, the Finkels had an elaborate funeral," Mrs. Frumkin said at dinner. "At the funeral, Gertie Finkel said, 'Well, she finally succeeded,' and soon left for Phoenix with her husband. Since Sonya killed herself, Isadore Finkel hasn't had another heart attack. The Finkels come to New York to visit every few months. I saw them a while ago, and they looked so gorgeous. It's no wonder. The cause of all their trouble was removed."

As Sylvia reached for her fourth serving of meat, potatoes, bread, and gravy, she said, "Ma, are you trying to tell me something?"

Yom Kippur, on Wednesday, October 11, was another bad day at the Frumkins'. Joyce was home again. That afternoon, Mrs. Frumkin had noticed that Sylvia was persistently biting her lower lip, and asked her whether she was getting any side effects from her medication. Sylvia, who hadn't heard her mother clearly, thought she had accused her of not taking her medication — something she had often failed to do in the past, with disastrous results. Sylvia got angry, grabbed her mother's arm, and twisted it. "Don't you dare talk to me about my medication!" she yelled. "I know what it is and when to take it!"

Joyce had been watching and had seen the look of pain on her mother's face. "You twisted your mother's arthritic arm, you blimp!" she shouted at Sylvia, stepping between her mother and her sister and comforting her mother.

"You think you're such a big shot!" Sylvia shouted at Joyce. "But who in this family went to medical-secretarial school? Who went to Music and Art? Me."

Sylvia had slept late on Yom Kippur, had gone to temple, and had fasted for several hours. At sundown, she began to make up for the few hours during which she hadn't eaten. She slurped her food down even more noisily than usual.

"Can't you leave Creedmoor there when you come home?" Mrs. Frumkin said.

"You're eating like a pig," Joyce said.

Sylvia picked up a bowl of potato salad that was on the dining-room table, raised it as if to throw it at Joyce, put it down, made a fist, walked over to her with a menacing look, and then went to her room. "I don't bring Creedmoor home, I come home to it!" she shouted, and she slammed the door. She took all the clothes out of her closet, searching for a blouse she wanted. When it was time to go back to Creedmoor, she refused to put any of the clothes back. Mrs. Frumkin told her that if she didn't pick her clothes up she would be punished. Her punishment would be that she would not be allowed to come home the following weekend. "Coming home means more to you than it does to me," Mrs. Frumkin said. Sylvia left all her clothes on the floor of her room.

Sylvia Frumkin and her mother spoke on the telephone several times during the next two days. On October 12, Sylvia pleaded to come home for the weekend. Usually, her mother gave in to her pleading. This time, she didn't. "Daddy says that you've got to learn that once in a while when we say something we mean it," Mrs. Frumkin said.

When Sylvia telephoned home on the thirteenth, her mother began the conversation by asking, "Honey, how are you?"

"Look, you don't want me home, so don't honey me," Sylvia said. "I'm not your honey." She hung up.

Sylvia called home on Saturday morning to see if her father was coming to pick her up. The Frumkins had been about to relent and take Sylvia home for the weekend, but their car needed new brake linings and some other work, and Mr. Frumkin had taken it to a mechanic to be fixed.

On Sunday, the Frumkins drove to Creedmoor and took Sylvia out for dinner at the Happy Robin. They made up. "It's not good to stay angry," Mrs. Frumkin said.

Sylvia Frumkin wasn't sorry she hadn't gone home for the weekend of the fourteenth and fifteenth. "I never have a relaxing time at home," she told one of the therapy aides on Saturday after she returned from a trip to a shopping center near Creedmoor. "I'm just glad I have grounds privileges, so that I can get off this awful ward."

⁊ ⁊ ⁊

Ward 043 had been a more tolerable place for Miss Frumkin when she was acutely psychotic and only partly aware of what she was saying and doing — half in the real world and half in an imagined world of television and movie stars and rock-and-roll singers. It was better to be the one who was begging others for food and cigarettes and coins than the one being begged. It was easier to be on the giving end of the punches than on the receiving end. In August and September, after Miss Frumkin had been stabilized on medication, she was eager to move on. The arrival of autumn made her realize how long she had been at Creedmoor. "I'd hoped to get out of here while it was still light in the morning," she said one day when she was awakened to October's 6:00 A.M. darkness. So many of the patients who had come to Clearview about the same time she did, or later, like Eileen O'Reilly, had left the ward. Miss Frumkin made no friends. A number of people who knew Miss Frumkin found that once she was no longer delusional, some of the engaging qualities that had beguiled Miss O'Reilly — her whimsy, her capriciousness, her way with words — left her. Although she usually stopped hitting people when she got "weller," she lashed out at them verbally. People who first met Miss Frumkin in October of 1978 met an aggressive, hypercritical, overtalkative know-it-all who made many remarks about others that seemed gratuitously unkind, and who was terribly abrupt. One minute, she would be talking to an acquaintance in the ward. The next minute, she would have lost interest in her, turned away, and said she would rather read a book or watch television.

Clearview's shabby conditions bothered her more that fall. One day, a group of women from Clearview went to the beauty shop in the Rehab Building to have their hair washed and set. A beautician said she had discovered that the first woman seated in the chair had lice. She and the other Clearview women were sent back to the ward. All the patients in the Clearview unit had to have their hair shampooed with Kwell. The idea of lice made Miss Frumkin shudder. That fall, she found more fault with the staff — especially with the 4:00-to-12:30 evening shift. They had always struck her as having a particularly uppity attitude toward patients. They often sat around reading their newspapers on chairs covered by white sheets. When a memo expressly forbidding this practice was sent around Creedmoor, they ignored it, and would warn some visitors not to sit down without first inspecting a chair, because "the patients are dirty." Some of the mahatas on the evening shift performed their duties unwillingly. They seemed to resent having to escort patients to the soda and snack machines in the central corridor during the prescribed hour after dinner allotted to the patients to use the machines, and seemed no less resentful of having to let patients make telephone calls. They were slow to leave their sheet-covered chairs to go to the television set, unlock the plastic screen, and turn the dial when patients asked to see a program on a different channel. They were in a hurry to get the patients to bed early — even the few patients, like Miss Frumkin, who wanted to stay up late. These mahatas had other interests, among them buying meat from a man who came around on their shift, parked his truck in back of N/4, and sold them pot roasts and steaks of unknown origin at prices well below those at the supermarket.

In the fall, Miss Frumkin easily became irritated by new patients who were as disturbed as she had been in the summer and who behaved accordingly. She fought with Isabelle Holzman, a young woman who had returned to Creedmoor after a couple of months away, because Miss Holzman took her clothes. She fought with a woman who took her chair. On the morning of October 25, before leaving for the Day Center, Miss Frumkin started to fight with a patient who had refused to move so that she could watch television. Therapy aides separated the two women, but not before Miss Frumkin had received a few small scratches on her face. That evening, a therapy aide wrote in her chart:

> At 8:10 P.M. after giving meds out I went to change channel on T.V. saying excuse first, & Sylvia started to scream & cursing & threatening. About 15 patients were sitting no one says anything but her, took my time and look for what I was asked to check about & then returned channel to original. By the time I was sitting in lunchroom there was one screaming in dormitory & there was Sylvia again at a patient, pulled off blanket & saying it was hers. Pt. is becoming very bizarre again & acting out. Nerves is at edge screaming & on top of her lungs. I told her plain she was not going to get her way, because she screams & yells.

Four days later, a therapy aide on the day shift also noted that Miss Frumkin was becoming more assaultive toward her peers. "It appears that pt. is waiting for an answer of whether or not she will be accepted at Transitional Services, and during this waiting period she is becoming agitated," the therapy aide wrote in her chart.

The therapy aide was right. October had been a difficult month for Miss Frumkin — a month of suspense, as she waited to hear from Transitional Services. On Thursday, November 2, she couldn't stand the suspense any longer. She walked over to Transitional Services and learned that she had not been accepted. The staff there believed that the pressure of Transitional's program would be too great. Later that day, after Miss Frumkin had returned to the ward, Dr. Sun happened to see her in the chart room. He noticed the lip-smacking, tongue-rolling, and lip-biting that Hermine Plotnick had seen and called to his attention a month and a half earlier. Dr. Sun now decided that these were, after all, symptomatic of tardive dyskinesia, and not just mannerisms, as he had first thought, and that he could arrest them if he reduced Miss Frumkin's medication. He lowered her medication immediately, from the 100 milligrams of Moban a day that she had been taking in recent weeks to 20 milligrams of Moban a day — 10 milligrams in the morning and 10 in the evening. He later said he would have preferred to lower the dose gradually — from 100 milligrams to 80 milligrams to 60 milligrams to 40 milligrams and only then to 20 milligrams — to lessen Miss Frumkin's chances of "decompensating" to her previous psychotic condition. He believed, however, that he had to lower it drastically because of the tardive dyskinesia.

⁊ ⁊ ⁊

On November 8 — the day after the New York State gubernatorial election, in which Miss Frumkin hadn't voted, and in which she hadn't expressed any interest since early June (she usually showed no interest in major events either at the hospital or in the outside world unless they directly affected her) — Miss Frumkin met with the ward social worker to discuss the bad news that she had been given by the counselor at Transitional Services. The only placement that Miss Frumkin and the Clearview treatment team had been working toward since her admission to Creedmoor on June 16 was Transitional Services. Now that this possibility had fallen through, they had to consider alternatives. Miss Frumkin and the social worker still agreed that it would be detrimental both for her and for her parents if she went home. Miss Frumkin wasn't keen on going to a halfway house: She had been asked to leave the first halfway house in which she had been placed, many years earlier, for having a messy room. She was terrified of winding up in an adult home. She told the social worker that what she wanted most was an apartment of her own. She also admitted that she didn't think she would be able to handle an apartment. "It would probably be too much for me," she said. "If I don't even make my bed at home, I doubt I could take care of an apartment." Looking back on November of 1978 from the perspective of February of 1979, the staff at Clearview believed that November was the month in which Miss Frumkin seemed to have the greatest intellectual insight into her predicament.

In November of 1978, after Miss Frumkin was turned down by Transitional Services, a social worker asked her how she felt about applying to the Clearview Motivation Center. Miss Frumkin said she had doubts about "the hotel," as the Motivation Center was invariably called, but that it would be better than the ward. The hotel's treatment team met on November 16 to consider Miss Frumkin. They decided that they would have to see how she did on the twenty milligrams of Moban for a whole month; only two weeks had gone by since the dose had been lowered. They agreed to consider her again at the end of the month. After being turned down at Transitional Services in early November, Miss Frumkin had extracted a consolation prize from the social worker: She was to be allowed to attend the typing workshop all day and could stop going to the Day Center.

Miss Frumkin's quarrels with her family intensified in November. Some years earlier, her parents had bought her a pretty fifty-dollar bedspread that was not washable and had to be dry-cleaned. Mrs. Frumkin had put it in a storage closet and had put a less expensive, less attractive, washable bedspread on Sylvia's bed. When Sylvia said she wanted to use her good spread ("What was the point in buying it?"), her mother said she couldn't use it because she never bathed and always threw the bedspread on the floor — and "dry-cleaning costs money." Mrs. Frumkin was upset by her younger daughter's sloth, her nail-picking, and her overeating. At the end of November, Sylvia weighed 180 pounds. "For thirty years, I've been nice to you," Harriet Frumkin told Sylvia one weekend in November. "Now I'm not going to be nice anymore." The tension at home increased when a four-day Thanksgiving weekend stretched into six days at home: Sylvia came home on Thursday, November 23, caught a bad cold, and was unable to return to Creedmoor until Wednesday, November 29. During those six days, she didn't get washed or dressed and didn't brush her teeth. She had also started to skip her medication on weekends.

The month of November at least ended more cheerfully for Miss Frumkin than it had begun. On Thursday, November 30, she was scheduled to be screened for the hotel. A month had gone by since Dr. Sun lowered her medication. He told the hotel treatment team that he had observed that her symptoms of tardive dyskinesia had been arrested, and that although she was demanding and manipulative, she was also rather calm, communicative, and realistic. He also said she wasn't a difficult management problem. Whether or not a patient was a management problem was a matter of some concern to the hotel treatment team, because the hotel staff was small: There were frequently only two therapy aides at the hotel per shift.

The Clearview Motivation Center's purpose was to assist

Clearview patients who no longer needed to be confined to a locked ward but could not yet be discharged directly to make the transition from the hospital to the community. The hotel not only met a real need, by improving the quality of life for those patients it admitted and by helping to release them, but also met a legal requirement. In 1975, the Supreme Court had decided in a landmark case that mental patients had to be kept in the least restrictive setting necessary for their well-being. Patients who didn't require confinement to locked wards were legally entitled to be housed in more open settings. The hotel team had met on the morning of November 30 to study Miss Frumkin's chart. That afternoon, the hotel treatment team and the ward treatment team met in the 043-044 chart room. The hotel's coordinator said that the members of the hotel team had seriously considered not accepting Miss Frumkin, since, in view of her history, they weren't optimistic about her chances of being discharged to the community, despite their best efforts. But, he went on to say, they had decided to accept her. "We'll try our hardest with Sylvia," he said. "At least we can provide her with a better environment than the ward."

After the coordinator had spoken, Mrs. Plotnick, who was at the meeting, said she wanted to thank the ward treatment team that had made it possible for Miss Frumkin to move from the ward to the hotel. In five and a half months at Creedmoor, Miss Frumkin had gone from being a helpless person who had to be almost continuously locked up in a seclusion room to being a person who could spend a full day in the typing workshop and be transferred to the hotel. It was perhaps indicative of the transience of Clearview's professional personnel that few of the people Mrs. Plotnick thanked on November 30, including the treatment-team leader, the social worker, and the psychologist, had been at Clearview when Miss Frumkin was admitted. Most of the departed personnel had transferred to other wards. Although Dr. Sun, who had admitted Miss Frumkin, was still there, he, too, would be leaving soon. In the summer of 1979, he was indicted for selling more than five thousand prescriptions of Valium and Tuinal at the private clinic in the Bronx where he worked part time. In September of 1979, he pleaded guilty to conspiring to distribute controlled substances without a legitimate medical purpose — a felony. In May of 1980, Dr. Sun was placed on probation for two years on the condition that he contribute 250 hours of community service in each of those years.

Mrs. Plotnick was as harshly critical of Creedmoor as the visitors to her unit and the patients. (The hospital's director, Dr. William L. Werner, was also a harsh critic of the institution.) Mrs. Plotnick decried Clearview's understaffing, its tawdry (and often dangerous) conditions, such as the lack of a padded seclusion room, and the many mistakes made there. One day in November when she was walking through one of the wards, she heard a mahata shout at an incontinent patient, "You're a dirty old thing!" She had recently been told by one of the treatment-team leaders that another mahata had said to a patient who had asked to watch a cartoon show on television, "You can't. I'm watching my favorite soap opera."

"Creedmoor should be so much better than it is, but it's a relatively safe place to be crazy," Mrs. Plotnick said after the meeting. "Sylvia Frumkin was much less likely to die from infection or malnutrition in Clearview than she would have been on the street. At the very least, we gave her asylum in the good sense of that word — a secure retreat."

When Miss Frumkin was called into the chart room and informed that she would be admitted to the hotel, she appeared joyful. "Thank heavens, knock on wood," she said. "The last time I was in the hotel, I made it. I went from the hotel to Transitional in February of 1977. Maybe I'll make it again."

⁄ ⁄ ⁄

Miss Frumkin was in a good mood when she moved to the Clearview hotel, at ten o'clock on December 4. The hotel was an attractive, sprawling two-story building of dark-red brick within easy walking distance of N/4. The hotel's residents lived in single or double rooms; there was a bathroom on each floor for men, and one for women. The room to which Miss Frumkin was assigned had two beds. Her spirits became even brighter when she learned that for the time being she would not have a roommate. Miss Frumkin often describes herself as a loner, and says forthrightly that she has no use for roommates. Not only can she not stand smoke but she likes to stay up later than most people and doesn't want to have to accommodate herself to other people's living patterns.

Miss Frumkin spent the weekend of the second and third of December at home. Her parents drove her back to Creedmoor on December 4 and helped her move the few things she had in the ward and a number of belongings from home to the hotel — some books, several changes of clothes, her guitar, a portable radio (a belated birthday gift from one of her mother's friends), and her blow dryer. As Sylvia unpacked, Mrs. Frumkin said, "You've made so much progress you're back at the hotel where you started two years ago." Sylvia Frumkin always hears what her mother says, but sometimes she decides to ignore her mother's thrusts. She preferred to dwell on the positive aspects of being in the hotel and out of the ward. Her room was austere — it was furnished with only the beds, two dressers, a closet, a washbasin, and a scatter rug — but it was preferable to a space in a dormitory. Testing the beds, Miss Frumkin said happily that both were real beds, with real box springs, and the mattresses and pillows had soft ticking, in contrast to the ward's hard beds and hard pillows. She made her choice and put clean sheets and a spread on the bed nearer the window, then arranged her set of Tolkien books on her dresser top. She liked the idea of being able to sleep until seven o'clock instead of six o'clock on weekdays and as late as she pleased on the weekends she didn't go home. She looked forward to signing out of the hotel in the morning, not having to return for a midafternoon count, and being able to stay out as late as ten-thirty without asking special permission.

One hotel rule that Miss Frumkin recalled from 1977 was that new residents had to stay at the hotel for ten days before they could go home. Miss Frumkin seemed pleased that she would not be able to go home on the weekend of the ninth and tenth of December. After spending a pleasant week at typing and a pleasant Saturday sleeping late, rereading *The Lord of the Rings,* and playing her guitar for the first time in over a year, Miss Frumkin went to church on Sunday morning. She had been going to a church near Creedmoor for the past several weeks without telling her parents, who would not have approved: They associated a number of Miss Frumkin's previous setbacks with religious conversions. She had been having religious dreams, which she also kept to herself. In some of her good dreams, she heard Christian music, with angels singing; in her nightmares, she saw demons. The Frumkins came to the hotel on the afternoon of Sunday, December 10, and took Sylvia to a small store near the hospital to buy her the first new clothes she had had in a year — except for the missing Peruvian poncho. They selected a four-piece polyester set consisting of black slacks, a black vest, a white blouse, and a tan jacket with black piping. When Sylvia looked around the store and found a black skirt that matched the set almost exactly, her parents bought her that, too. The clothes were size 18, but they were well-cut and flattering, and she was happy to have them. Sicker or weller, she often expressed her resentment at having to wear other people's old clothes.

⸙ ⸙ ⸙

The following week was also an agreeable one for Miss Frumkin. On December 11, she took a typing test and scored thirty-five words a minute with fourteen errors — an improvement. For the past several weeks, she had been earning small sums of money stuffing envelopes, affixing labels to envelopes, and typing a few envelopes. On December 13, there was a Christmas party at the typing workshop. The class had the whole day off from typing. The party began in the morning, with games like musical chairs, pin the button on Santa's nose, Simon says, and charades. A few clients cried and refused to play any games, but Miss Frumkin participated with enthusiasm, as she had at the typing workshop's Halloween party, when she enjoyed bobbing for apples and playing pin the stem on the pumpkin.

The tables at the back of the typing room had been covered with festive Christmas and Chanukah paper tablecloths, on which a banquet had been laid out. There were platters of fried chicken and bowls of coleslaw, potato chips, pretzels, pickles, M&M's, Hershey's Kisses, and pitchers of punch. Miss Frumkin ate more than anyone else. "I'll diet after Christmas," she said to a client who had commented, "Six handfuls of M&M's, Sylvia, six handfuls."

Miss Frumkin seemed preoccupied after she had finished eating. A talent show had been planned for the early afternoon. She was to play her guitar. She bit her fingernails, she twiddled her fingers, and she worried that there were fewer people present at the Christmas party than there had been at the Halloween party. She kept repeating that she hadn't played her guitar in a long time and had been up practicing until two o'clock in the morning and would have stayed up all night if a mahata on night duty at the hotel hadn't made her go to bed. She plucked at the guitar strings while the other guests were eating lunch. She was the first to perform. "Wish me luck," she said to the audience before she started to play "White Christmas." She occasionally stopped playing to shush those members of the audience who in her opinion weren't giving her their undivided attention. Her second song was "The Little Drummer Boy," which she seemed to find more difficult than her first selection. She made a mistake, asked "Can we please start over?," started over, made another mistake, and asked the audience's permission to begin again. Finally, one of the clients said, "Enough is enough, Sylvia." She then got through the song without any serious mistakes. In September Miss Frumkin had asked Mrs. Gruen if she could be Santa Claus at the Christmas party. She had been given the part. She put on a Santa Claus mask, took a seat at the back of the room next to a box full of wrapped gifts, and was a jovial Santa Claus. She asked each client in the line to tell Santa how she'd been doing in typing and what she wanted for Christmas. Santa Frumkin handed out Christmas cards that had been crayoned and pasted by a local troop of Camp Fire Girls and small bottles of cologne that had been donated by a large cosmetics manufacturer. Her stint as Santa Claus over, she took off the Santa Claus mask and asked Mrs. Gruen, "Are we going to have an Easter party?" Mrs. Gruen told her it was not the time to worry about Easter — it was time for the group to sing Christmas and Chanukah songs. After the singing, the party was over.

The following day, during the typing workshop's lunch break, Miss Frumkin walked to a beauty parlor near Creedmoor to get her hair cut. She had decided that Huntington was too far to travel, even for Jason. The beauty shop near Creedmoor was convenient. She liked Heidi, the young woman who cut her hair, because Heidi was friendly and also seemed to believe her when she said that she worked at Creedmoor as a secretary. That evening, the residents of Clearview's hotel were going to dinner in Manhasset, at the home of Creedmoor's supervisor of volunteer services. Creedmoor's large bus had been reserved to transport forty hotel residents and several members of the hotel staff to and from the party. Miss Frumkin put on her new blouse, vest, pants, and jacket. The night was cold, so she also put on a brown winter coat that one of the volunteers at Jewish services had recently given her. The patients rode to Manhasset in silence. The fifteen-minute ride from Creedmoor to Manhasset turned into a forty-five-minute ride, because the bus driver had had a few drinks for the road and lost his way.

The supervisor of volunteer services' elegant Tudor house had been beautifully decorated for the holidays. The hotel residents were greeted, assisted in taking off their coats, and escorted to the recreation room, where they were seated at small tables. A dinner of barbecued chicken and barbecued ribs, salad, rolls, apple cider, and a selection of cakes, cookies, and pies was served to them. The hotel residents ate in silence. After dinner, they went upstairs and sat down in the living room, where a floor-to-ceiling tree trimmed with handmade ornaments and strings of lights sparkled prettily, and where a Juilliard student had just started to play the piano. Next, two Creedmoor volunteers sang and played the guitar. Then the hotel residents were asked if they wanted to sing solos. Miss Frumkin was the first to say she did. She sang "It Came Upon the Midnight Clear." Two of the other hotel residents also sang solos. There was some group caroling, in which only a few hotel residents joined, and then it was time to reboard the bus. The hotel residents thanked the host as they filed out the front door. They boarded the bus and rode back to the hotel in silence. Over the following months, they often told their host that they had had a lovely time at his Christmas party. No one would have known it from watching them that evening. No one would have known it from seeing photographs that Mrs. Plotnick had taken of many of the hotel residents during the evening. A friend of Mrs. Plotnick's who saw the snapshots said that they brought to mind a line spoken by a character in a play she had seen many years earlier: "Wherever I go, I take myself with me, and that always spoils it." There wasn't one photograph that showed a person who was talking or smiling.

⁄ ⁄ ⁄

In December, Miss Frumkin had appeared reasonably cheerful: The combination of moving to the hotel and the busyness of the holiday season seemed to contribute to her good humor. A week or so before Christmas, Harriet Frumkin had given Sylvia her bankbook. It was the first time that Miss Frumkin had had her bankbook in her possession since she surrendered it to Stephanie Fulton in July. Now that she was earning some money at the typing workshop, she went to the bank several times a week. She deposited the small sums she received every two weeks from the typing workshop, and she deposited her weekly allowance. She withdrew several dollars every few days for her expenses, taking care to keep her balance above two hundred dollars. She spent most of her money on food. In January, she became increasingly nervous and unhappy. She became very critical of the hotel. She complained that the mahatas who walked through the halls of the hotel knocking on the doors of the rooms at seven o'clock to say it was time to get up were grouchy. She found fault with the activities at the hotel. She had formerly enjoyed participating in bingo games that were held there some evenings, but she now told the hostesses from the churches that sponsored the bingo games that the prizes weren't as good as they used to be, and she also told them they should bring more potato chips and fewer pretzels. She confided to one acquaintance that she no longer felt comfortable playing bingo; she thought it might be a pagan activity, a form of gambling inappropriate to Christians. Her acquaintance told her not to worry — bingo was played in churches.

In December, whenever Miss Frumkin spoke to the members of the hotel team about her discharge, she spoke of eventually returning to Transitional Services. On January 10, 1979, during a regularly scheduled meeting of the hotel staff and its residents, Miss Frumkin suddenly informed the hotel team that she was no longer planning to go back to Transitional. She told the hotel team that Transitional Services had some advantages over the hotel. At Transitional, wakeup time was at seven-thirty instead of seven. The food was better, and the people behind the food-service counters treated you like a human being. The personnel at Transitional Services — with a few exceptions — were friendlier. At Transitional, you could lock the door to your room, and four women, at most, shared a bathroom, instead of eight or ten. And the residents of Transitional were people who had been discharged from the hospital and were better off financially, because they could draw S.S.I., whereas the hotel residents were still Creedmoor patients and couldn't. But, she went on to tell the hotel team, Transitional Services was still on the Creedmoor grounds. It was a structured program. You usually had a roommate there. She said she was fed up with living on the hospital grounds and with being regulated. She wanted to live alone in the community — in her own apartment. The members of the team told Miss Frumkin, as tactfully as they could, that her record at Transitional Services and at the hotel indicated that a supervised setting was a more realistic living arrangement for her. They reminded her that her room at the hotel was a mess and that she resisted getting out of bed every morning. They told her politely but firmly that she wasn't ready for an apartment. Miss Frumkin repeated that nothing but her own apartment would suit her. The members of the team said they would talk to her again in a few weeks.

In late January, Miss Frumkin appeared lazier, more tense, and more argumentative. At the typing workshop, she talked too much and was so anxious that when she was given five envelopes to type at one time she made many errors. When Mrs. Gruen and Mrs. Wilcox gave her only one envelope at a time, she felt humiliated, because all the other clients were given five at a time. She picked at her fingers more — in typing, at the hotel, and at home. Some days, she bought special contour bandages and spent ten straight hours taping her fingers so that she couldn't pick at them. The following day, she would undo ten hours of labor in fifteen minutes by unwrapping the bandages. Not only didn't she want to get out of bed or clean her room, she didn't want to wash. The hotel staff reminded her to take showers when her body odor became offensive to others. Miss Frumkin was never popular with her peers, because she was always giving advice to others and rejecting it from them, but she became even less popular in late January. She monopolized resident group meetings at the hotel with lengthier and lengthier monologues. At one group meeting, she talked for twenty minutes about dieting. She said she was going to buy a box of Ayds vanilla caramels, because she didn't like the taste of them, instead of buying a box of chocolate-mint Ayds, which she did like and ate as if they were candy, but she then said she probably wouldn't buy Ayds in any flavor. Instead, she would join Overeaters Anonymous, Weigh of Life, or one of the other support groups for compulsive eaters, but she wasn't sure when. In the meantime, when she went to McDonald's and ordered hot-fudge sundaes with extra fudge she was hurt when she heard people in line behind her saying that McDonald's would be doing her a favor if they refused to sell her sundaes. As she was lamenting the fact that she weighed 185, an outspoken patient who had had enough of listening to her said, "The more you talk about dieting, the less you do about it, so why don't you shut up?"

The following evening, Miss Frumkin said she hadn't had any eggnog over the holidays, and went to the delicatessen to buy some. A man at the hotel had given her money to get him a sandwich and a soda. When she returned with a quart of eggnog and his order, she went to his room and invited him to eat in her room. As he ate his sandwich slowly, he watched and listened to her gulp down the whole quart in a few minutes, burping between swallows. She explained that she had had to buy a whole quart of eggnog because there were no half pints or pints of eggnog for sale at the delicatessen. The man had a girlfriend in the hotel who was due to go to visit her sister the following weekend. Miss Frumkin suggested he take her out that Saturday night. The man agreed. Two days later, he reneged. An older woman who had had the job of working in the hotel snack bar every evening was about to be discharged from Creedmoor. Miss Frumkin knew that the job paid a dollar an evening, and applied for it. She was told she was too sloppy to handle it. The job was given to another young woman.

In late January, Miss Frumkin told her acquaintances at the typing workshop that she was getting more and more obsessive. She had noticed that she was counting the number of steps she took when she walked from the hotel to the dining room, which was in a nearby building, and that she was counting the brushstrokes when she brushed her teeth — on the rare days that she did brush her teeth. She also spent two hours a day on her budget, poring over her figures, because she was always three or four cents off in her calculations.

⸙ ⸙ ⸙

Voluntary patients at Creedmoor are supposed to be given a form to sign at least every 120 days to indicate their wish to remain in the hospital. On January 24, Miss Frumkin was given the form and didn't hesitate to scrawl her name on it. If she had asked for her release then — or, for that matter, if she had asked for her release in September, October, November, or December — she would have been discharged, "against medical advice." Clearview's psychiatrists believed that Miss Frumkin could benefit from a continued stay at the hotel, to prepare for her gradual reentry into the community, or they would have already discharged her; but they would not have contested her request for a release if she had asked for one. The psychiatrists would not have wanted to go to court to testify that Miss Frumkin was dangerous to herself or others, because she clearly had coping skills in the fall of 1978 and the winter of 1979 that she had lacked when she was admitted to the hospital the previous June 16.

Five days after signing the voluntary form, Miss Frumkin had a demonic nightmare. Afterward, she told an employee at the hotel that she had got down on her knees and had found Christ again. The next day, she told an acquaintance at the typing workshop that she had had enough of everything and that she wanted to make a clean break with things. The acquaintance wasn't sure what Miss Frumkin meant. She knew how volatile and changeable Miss Frumkin was, and knew that she took a certain pleasure in being mysterious.

On the night of Tuesday, February 6, it began to snow in New York City. The snow fell softly and steadily all through the night. Miss Frumkin put her nightgown on that evening, but she didn't go to sleep. She stayed up all night reading the Bible, rustling the pages of the New Testament noisily. For the first time in months, Miss Frumkin heard voices. The voices told her to leave the hospital immediately.

At seven o'clock the next morning, when a hotel mahata knocked on her door to tell her it was "that time again," Miss Frumkin didn't dally. It was still snowing. She put on her new black skirt. "Ladies don't wear slacks," she said to an acquaintance at the hotel, although she had worn nothing but slacks for months. She put on a blouse, a jacket, a vest, a coat, and a pair of boots. She took her big pocketbook with her. She went to get her morning medication — the ten milligrams of Moban — and walked out of the hotel. Around ten o'clock that evening, a hotel mahata on the 4:00-to-12:30 shift realized that she hadn't seen Miss Frumkin since coming on duty. Hotel residents often stayed out in the community until ten-thirty, so she wasn't worried. At eleven, when Miss Frumkin still hadn't returned, the hotel mahata called Irving and Harriet Frumkin to ask if Sylvia had by any chance come home. She hadn't. The mahata then called the Safety Department to report her missing. She made out an incident report saying that Miss Frumkin had gone on a leave without consent. Harriet Frumkin called Joyce and several friends to ask if they had heard from Sylvia that day. They hadn't.

On the morning of February 8, Miss Frumkin had still not returned to the hotel. The hotel's social worker called Mrs. Frumkin; Sylvia still hadn't come home, either. The social worker then called the typing workshop and asked Mrs. Wilcox if Miss Frumkin had been there on February 7. Mrs. Wilcox said she hadn't. She explained to the social worker that under normal circumstances she would have telephoned the hotel to ask where Miss Frumkin was, but that so many people were absent on the seventh because of the heavy snow that she hadn't called the numerous absentees. The Frumkins were frantic. They telephoned the Missing Persons Squad and spent most of the day on the telephone with their friends. They tried to recall what Sylvia had told them about her life at Creedmoor in recent weeks. They remembered that she had spoken of wanting to have lunch with Edith, one of the out-patients who attended the typing workshop. They called Edith at home. She hadn't heard from Sylvia. The Frumkins remembered that Sylvia had complained that a Creedmoor patient named Larry had been bothering her for dates. The social worker called Larry's ward. He hadn't left the grounds on the seventh or the eighth, and knew nothing about Sylvia's disappearance.

On the morning of the ninth, the Frumkins learned from a detective in the Missing Persons Squad that Sylvia had withdrawn two hundred dollars from her bank on February 7. The balance in her account was now only thirty-four dollars. The detectives told Mrs. Frumkin that Sylvia hadn't been able to withdraw that sum, because the thirty-four dollars consisted of checks she had recently deposited, which hadn't yet cleared. The knowledge that Sylvia had taken two hundred dollars with her on her flight was anything but reassuring to her parents.

The Frumkins and the Clearview staff spent some time that Friday speculating on the reasons for Sylvia's sudden departure. Some of the staff believed that after her meeting with the hotel team on January 10, when she told the team that she wanted an apartment and was informed that she wasn't ready for one, she had felt thwarted. After a month, she had assimilated the news, had felt she was at the end of her rope, and had taken off. Some people conjectured that she might have been more hurt than she let on when the man at the hotel declined to take her out and when she was bypassed for the job in the hotel snack bar. Mrs. Plotnick believed that by early February Miss Frumkin was beginning to feel the effects of the drastic reduction in her medication that had taken place in early November. Mrs. Plotnick had learned from observing many patients over the years that the majority of patients felt well for the first month after they stopped taking their medication: The medication's unpleasant side effects ceased, and their psychotic symptoms didn't reappear, because there was a considerable amount of medication left in their systems. As a result, many patients thought they hadn't needed the medication in the first place. During the second month off medication, many patients began to decompensate. By the third month, many were psychotic. Because Miss Frumkin was so heavy, she probably had a good deal of medication stored in her fatty tissues, so it was not surprising that it had taken her three months to hear voices.

On the evening of Friday, February 9, the doctor covering the Clearview hotel formally discharged Miss Frumkin from Creedmoor. She was a voluntary patient who had been missing almost seventy-two hours. He wouldn't be at the hotel on Saturday, when she would have been gone for precisely seventy-two hours — he wouldn't be back at the hospital before Monday — and regulations required that voluntary patients be discharged as soon as they had been gone that long. If Sylvia Frumkin returned before the seventy-two hours were up, his discharge could always be voided by the doctor on call on Saturday. After the doctor covering the hotel discharged Miss Frumkin, he telephoned the Frumkins and the Safety Department.

Not long after the doctor called the Frumkins to tell them that Sylvia had been discharged from Creedmoor, their telephone rang again. Mr. Frumkin answered the telephone. A man was on the line. His name was George Klopfer, and he assured Irving Frumkin that his daughter was safe. Klopfer and his wife, Nellie, had taken Miss Frumkin into their home in 1975, at another critical time in her life, and they had agreed to do so again when she turned up at their house, in upstate New York, on February 7. The Klopfers were born-again Christians. They believed that Miss Frumkin was possessed by demons. The next morning, Miss Frumkin telephoned her parents. She sounded very happy. She called them several times over the next few days. Each time she called, she said, "With Jesus Christ, everything is going to work out fine."

III

The Illness Is Stronger Than I Am

Eleven

When Sylvia Frumkin was born in Brooklyn on May 5, 1948, her parents were both forty. Irving Frumkin was born in a village in Belorussia, to Morris and Yenta Frumkin, who were first cousins. He was the third of five children: He had two older sisters, Molly and Bertha, and two younger brothers, Julius and Hyman. Morris Frumkin was in the lumber business. In 1911, shortly after the birth of his fifth child, a big lumber contract fell through and the business went bankrupt. Yenta Frumkin had three brothers who had gone to the United States ten years earlier. One brother, Reuben Schor, had become a wealthy restaurateur in Brooklyn. Morris Frumkin left Russia for the United States in 1911 with the conviction that he, too, would prosper there and would be able to send for his family in two or three years. Reuben gave Morris Frumkin a job as a waiter in one of his restaurants. By the spring of 1914, Morris had saved enough money to send for his family. In those days, small banks in such sections of Brooklyn as Williamsburg and East New York, where immigrants like Morris Frumkin settled, acted as travel agents for men who wanted to send to the old country for their families. Morris Frumkin gave a bank five hundred dollars for ship passage for his wife and children. The bank declared bankruptcy a few months after he had paid for the tickets. Before he could earn enough money to buy tickets for his family on another ship, the First World War broke out. For some years, travel between Russia and the United States came to a standstill.

From 1911 to 1918, Yenta Frumkin supported herself and her children by working as a seamstress. They were poor, but the hardships they experienced were relatively minor. In 1918, civil war broke out in Belorussia. For the next three years, there was a severe food shortage in the area, and the family had nothing but potato sacks to wrap around their feet during the bitter Russian winters. In 1921, Morris Frumkin returned to Russia and made arrangements for his family to immigrate to America. They reached Ellis Island in February of 1923. Morris Frumkin had disliked waiting on tables, but he had kept at it for his family's sake. Three years after Morris brought his family over, Reuben Schor, who was fond of Yenta, his only sister, lent the Frumkins a thousand dollars so that they could open a small grocery store in East New York. Yenta and Morris Frumkin ran the store until their retirement, twenty years later.

Irving Frumkin arrived in America speaking fluent Yiddish (the language spoken in the Frumkin home) and passable Russian. Despite the various pogroms, the First World War, the Russian civil war, and all the accompanying political turmoil, he had received some schooling and was proficient in such subjects as algebra and geometry. Because his English was almost nonexistent, he was put in the third grade of the local public school in East New York. He dropped out after a few weeks and went to work; he eventually earned a high-school diploma by attending night classes. As a teen-ager, he held a series of low-paying factory jobs. After seeing at first hand the perilous working conditions and meager wages paid in the factories, he quit a twenty-cent-an-hour job as a power-press operator and went to work as a journalist at a Yiddish newspaper. In 1937, while Irving Frumkin was still living at home with his parents, in East New York, he met Harriet Wilder.

Harriet Wilder Frumkin is not forthright about her age. She would prefer to have her family and friends believe that she was only thirty-five when Sylvia Frumkin was born. She left the space for her age blank on Sylvia's birth certificate, and she would like to carry the secret of her age to her grave. Mrs. Frumkin has already told her oldest daughter, Joyce, that when she dies she wants just the date of her death inscribed on her tombstone — not the date of her birth.

Harriet Frumkin's parents, Minna Eskolsky and Saul Wilder, both came to the United States as teen-agers, from the Ukraine. They met on the Lower East Side. Saul Wilder earned a modest living as a furrier. The Wilders' daughter, Harriet, was born on May 1, 1908; their son, Benjamin, was born on July 23, 1916. Both Wilder children were gifted. Harriet Wilder started taking painting classes when she was eight. When she was twelve, she started giving art lessons to younger children on the Lower East Side, and later, after the Wilders moved to East New York, she gave lessons there. When she was fifteen, she was offered a scholarship to an art institute in Boston. She was unable to accept it, because her mother wouldn't countenance her living alone in a strange city — a fact she has never ceased to regret. After graduating from high school, Harriet Wilder went to a business college for a year and then went to work. The money she earned working as a secretary, as a free-lance illustrator for several magazines, and as an art teacher helped to put her younger brother through college during the Depression. After Benjamin Wilder finished college, he went into the army. When the war ended, he attended graduate school and became a prominent scientist.

Minna Eskolsky Wilder was the oldest of nine children and was the first person in her immediate family to come to the United States. She stayed with relatives after her arrival and worked as a seamstress to support herself and to earn money to send for the other members of the family. First, she brought over her brother Simon. Minna and Simon Eskolsky worked and saved, and eventually brought over their brother Harvey, their parents, and their six sisters — Lottie, Jessie, Goldie, Vera, Mona, and Helen. Minna Eskolsky Wilder has been described by her son and daughter as the family matriarch. Jessie, Goldie, and Mona married and had families and led independent lives, but Minna dominated the lives of Harvey (who remained a bachelor), Lottie (a spinster), and Vera, who became severely depressed as a young woman after her fiancé left her. Vera Eskolsky was hospitalized at Pilgrim State, New York's largest hospital for the mentally ill; she died there, of tuberculosis, in 1948.

Minna Eskolsky Wilder also tried to run the lives of her husband and their two children, and, according to her son, she succeeded in two cases out of three. Saul Wilder, a weak, submissive man, took refuge from his domineering wife in the fur shop he set up in the basement of the tenement building where the Wilders lived. (Minna's mother, Jaritza, was also a domineering woman. Her husband's refuge had been the synagogue.) Benjamin Wilder describes himself as his mother's son: He was as tough as she was, stood up to her as a young man, left Brooklyn after finishing college, married, moved away, and did not return home more than once or twice a year to visit. According to Benjamin Wilder, his sister was victimized by their mother. Harriet Wilder Frumkin, now a short, plain woman of seventy-three who colors her gray hair brown and almost always wears polyester pants suits, was an attractive young girl. She had several admirers, but Minna Wilder found fault with them and scared them off. She wanted to keep Harriet under her control, even though she always favored her assertive son over her submissive daughter. Minna Wilder made all of Harriet's clothes; she didn't let her have a store-bought dress until her high-school graduation. She didn't teach her daughter to use a sewing machine, however. Harriet Wilder was encouraged to be dependent; she never learned how to swim or how to drive a car.

In 1937, Harriet Wilder was introduced to Irving Frumkin by a friend of a friend of her brother's. Irving Frumkin was different from her other suitors. The others had been nice-looking, refined, and interested in the arts. Irving Frumkin was a short man with ordinary features. He was interested in nothing but politics and journalism. He dressed and ate sloppily, his hair was always messy, and he was a nonstop talker. Harriet Wilder and Irving Frumkin went out for a year and then stopped seeing each other. One day about a year later, Harriet was jostled in a crowded subway. "Stop pushing," she said to the person who had shoved her — who proved to be Irving Frumkin. He came over to visit her that evening; they started going out again. Early in 1939, Frumkin proposed marriage. Harriet accepted his proposal. "I was taken with his idealism," she said recently. "I thought he was the champion of the working class, and I was attracted by his sincerity and his high-mindedness." Several of Harriet Wilder's relatives attribute her decision to marry Irving Frumkin to the low sense of self-esteem that had been instilled in her by her mother and to her fear of becoming an old maid: She was over thirty when Frumkin proposed. Minna Wilder seemed to take a liking to Frumkin, and was less critical of him than she had been of her daughter's previous admirers, perhaps because he kowtowed to her. "When she said it was day, Irving said it was day, even if it was midnight," Benjamin Wilder recalls. "Argumentative as Irving was — and is — with everyone else, he took a subdued tone with Minna, and convinced her that she was gaining a son instead of losing a daughter. Irving genuinely liked my mother, and he was good to her all her life." In her later years, Minna Wilder always told her daughter that Irving Frumkin was much too good for her.

Harriet Wilder and Irving Frumkin were married on April 2, 1939, a month before her thirty-first birthday. After their return from a brief honeymoon, they set up housekeeping in a three-room apartment in East New York, just around the corner from the Wilders and three blocks from the Frumkins. Harriet Frumkin stopped working as an illustrator after her marriage, but she continued to do secretarial work and to give art lessons. She gave up her job as a secretary when she became pregnant with her first child. The child, a girl, was born on September 29, 1942, after a difficult delivery; she was named Joyce, after Minna Wilder's mother, Jaritza, who had died six months earlier. Soon after Joyce Frumkin learned to talk, it was apparent that she had some of her uncle's, her grandmother's, and her great-grandmother's strong character.

Joyce was a pretty, blond child and an easy one to bring up: She was good-natured, bright, and artistic. She started to do watercolors when she was six. Irving Frumkin doted on Joyce. He was constantly taking photographs of her and showing them off to his newspaper acquaintances, many of whom also saw her in person. Some of Joyce's earliest memories are of sitting on her father's shoulders when he covered parades in the mid-forties. Joyce admired her formidable grandmother Minna more than her Uncle Benjamin did, perhaps because she was a generation removed from Minna. When she came home after school and found her mother giving art lessons, she either got out her own paints or walked to her grandmother's house. Grandma Minna was an excellent cook and enjoyed spoiling her first grandchild.

After Joyce's birth, Harriet Frumkin's obstetrician advised her not to risk another pregnancy, and Irving Frumkin didn't want to have a second child. Mrs. Frumkin was determined to have another child, however — preferably a daughter. She was fond of her younger brother, but she had always been sorry that she hadn't had a sister, and she wanted Joyce to have one. She was delighted when she became pregnant in 1947, and delighted that the baby, born in May of 1948, was a girl; the baby was named Sylvia, after Harriet's father, Saul, who had died in 1943. Joyce, who was almost six when Sylvia was born, thought of her little sister as her baby. A photograph in the living room of the Frumkins' present home shows Joyce holding her infant sister as if she were a cherished doll. Sylvia was never to accompany her father to parades. By late 1947, Yiddish newspapers were losing circulation, and Mr. Frumkin lost his job. In 1948, he went to work for a bottling company in Brooklyn. He stayed with that company until it declared bankruptcy, in 1970. Harriet Frumkin was relieved when her husband took a job with regular hours, but since 1948 Irving Frumkin has been a bitter man. Just as his wife has lamented for over half a century the possible career she gave up as an artist, he has spent the last thirty years bemoaning his lost career as a journalist.

Joyce Frumkin started first grade in East New York in September of 1948, a few months after Irving Frumkin gave up his journalistic career. According to several of his relatives and acquaintances, he began to live his life through his older daughter. Joyce excelled at school. She brought home straight A's. Her father gloried in her achievements, but he was never quite satisfied with them and always put pressure on her to do even better. Joyce recalls that when she brought home a ninety-eight percent, her father would ask her, "Where's the other two percent?"

After the Second World War, East New York turned increasingly black and Puerto Rican. In July of 1952, the Frumkins moved to a four-room garden apartment in Beechhurst, a middle-middle-class section of Queens. The apartment had two large bedrooms. For Joyce Frumkin, the transition from fourth grade in Brooklyn to fifth grade in Queens was smooth. She made new friends easily, and she continued to get straight A's. Although Sylvia was only four at the time of the move and hadn't yet started school, she didn't adjust easily to the change. As a little girl, Sylvia was slender and had light-brown hair. She was precocious, like

Joyce. She walked early and she talked early. She talked incessantly, not only to her family but also to four or five imaginary friends, one of whom seemed to be special to her; his name was Grayson. If Mrs. Frumkin had any fault to find with Sylvia, it was that she was overtalkative, but when she mentioned this to a pediatrician he advised her not to worry. He told her that some children were just chatterboxes.

Sylvia gave up her imaginary friends when she started kindergarten, in 1953, but she complained that she had difficulty making real friends. The children she liked didn't seem to like her. She couldn't understand why. She was accepted only by children she called "the underdogs," and always felt like an underdog herself. Joyce understood some of the reasons for her sister's inability to make friends. Sylvia tried to latch on to other children, saying, "If you're going to be my friend, you can't be anyone else's," and thereby alienated them.

Sometimes Sylvia came home from school saying that a boy had hit her — one day it was Michael, one day it was Gary. Mrs. Frumkin would call Gary's mother to complain. Gary would deny having hit Sylvia. His mother would say, "My Gary wouldn't do a thing like that. He's a little gentleman, and he's always saying that Sylvia is one of the smartest girls in the class." Mrs. Frumkin would back off. Perhaps, after a friendly chat, Gary would start to take art lessons from Mrs. Frumkin. Other mothers were less cordial to Mrs. Frumkin when she called. "Why don't you put your daughter in a glass cage?" one woman asked her after her son had been wrongly accused of hitting Sylvia.

On a number of occasions, Sylvia's behavior was oddly provocative. One Saturday morning, Sylvia, Joyce, Mrs. Frumkin, a friend of Mrs. Frumkin's, and the friend's son, Fred, went to a neighborhood supermarket. Sylvia and Fred were then six or seven years old. Joyce, who was about thirteen, was charged with watching them on the sidewalk while their mothers shopped for groceries. There was a candy store next to the supermarket. Joyce told Sylvia and Fred that she was going in to buy some bubble gum and would be right back. Two minutes later, Joyce, Mrs. Frumkin, and Fred's mother could hear Fred screaming. All three came running out. While Fred yelled, Sylvia stood on the sidewalk quietly holding a doll she had brought along from home. After Fred stopped sobbing, his mother asked him what had happened. He told her that while he and Sylvia were standing on the sidewalk Sylvia had suddenly hit him over the head with her doll. Sylvia didn't deny it, so Mrs. Frumkin asked her why she had done that. "I knew Fred was going to hit me, so I was hitting him back first," Sylvia answered. Mrs. Frumkin reprimanded Joyce for leaving the two young children by themselves.

Whereas Joyce had received straight A's in grade school, Sylvia got an occasional B. She became angry when Mr. Frumkin said, "When Joyce was in first grade, she got a ninety-eight percent, and you got a ninety-six." She became equally angry when she brought home a seventy in math, her worst subject, and her father didn't comment. "You're not asking me for the missing thirty percent because you think that's the best I can do," she said. Joyce was always dressed well, in new clothes that fitted her properly. Sylvia was often dressed in ill-fitting hand-me-downs from Joyce. Her classmates made fun of her appearance. Mrs. Frumkin saw nothing wrong with passing clothes down from big sister to little sister. She and her husband were from poor families in which such a practice was regarded as sensible. Joyce was as neat as Sylvia was untidy. Mrs. Frumkin remembers that it was always easy to tell which half of the girls' bedroom was whose without asking. Joyce was usually the protective older sister and cleaned up both sides of the room, but Sylvia resented her. Sometimes she would give her arm a painful twist, just as she would sometimes pinch her mother or slap her father. She tried to compete with Joyce, but she viewed the competition as a losing battle. "Joyce is the top of the totem pole and I'm the bottom," Sylvia often said.

Joyce Frumkin took painting lessons and, later, classes in sculpture at an art school in Brooklyn. To outdo her, Sylvia said she wanted to go to an art school in Manhattan. When she was seven, she was accepted by the art school, and she studied there for the next seven years. When she was too young to travel alone, her father drove her into Manhattan every Saturday from Queens. He seemed eager to give his daughters some of the things of which he had been deprived by the circumstances of his life. One year while Sylvia was studying drawing at the art school, a cousin of hers who lived near the Frumkins in Queens was taking a pottery class in Manhattan. Irving Frumkin offered to drive both girls to and from the city. After a few Saturdays, the cousin told her mother that the car rides were unbearable. Sylvia decided where her cousin was to sit, she dominated the conversation, and she threatened to throw up whenever she felt she wasn't the center of attention. Mr. Frumkin always carried a bag in the car for her to use if she did throw up. The cousin soon chose to travel to Manhattan on Saturdays by subway and bus. One stormy Saturday, a friend of the Frumkins called up and was surprised to learn from Mrs. Frumkin that Mr. Frumkin was on his way into Manhattan with Sylvia. When she suggested that the art lesson wasn't worth the drive in such inclement weather, Mrs. Frumkin said, "You don't seem to understand. The lesson is important. We've paid for it."

Sylvia was artistically gifted, but not greatly so, and she decided that she didn't really care for drawing and painting. She told her parents she would prefer to take lessons in voice or guitar. Her mother said that since she was an art teacher, it would be more sensible for Sylvia to study art. Harriet Frumkin rarely had to tell Sylvia to do her homework, but she often had to tell her to get out her easel. "What's the good of painting when I'll never paint as well as you do?"

Sylvia asked her mother. Although she once painted some respectable landscapes, she refuses even to touch paints today.

The brightest sixth-graders in New York City's public schools are offered an opportunity to enter special seventh-grade rapid-advance classes, from which they can go directly into ninth grade after one year. Joyce Frumkin had easily done three years of junior high school in two years, and had gone on to a high school in Queens. She had been an officer of the high-school honor society, an editor of the high-school newspaper, and a member of the cheering squad. When she graduated from high school, in 1959, twenty-fifth in a class of several hundred, she was awarded two prizes. Joyce had applied to a number of colleges and had been accepted by all of them. In the late 1950s, Mr. Frumkin's annual income was about seven thousand dollars a year. Joyce chose to attend a women's college in upstate New York, which cost two thousand dollars a year. It was her first choice, and it had offered her the largest scholarship. She was glad to get away from home and to meet young women from "better" families. She worked hard to get rid of her Brooklyn accent, she made friends, and she had an active social life.

Sylvia, whose IQ was 138 when it was tested in grade school, was put into a seventh-grade rapid-advance class in the fall of 1960, just as Joyce had been six years earlier, but in junior high school Sylvia's troubles with other children became worse. Joyce was reasonably athletic, and had enjoyed her summers at camp, first as a camper, later as a junior counselor and a counselor. Sylvia was clumsy and poorly coordinated. She couldn't learn to swim, skate, jump rope, ride a bike, or throw a ball. She didn't like day camp as a young girl and never became a counselor. As a child, Sylvia had been small-boned and delicate-looking. She grew suddenly, reaching what was to be her full height — five feet four inches — at the age of eleven. From then on, she appeared awkward and unattractive. She was nearsighted and had to wear thick glasses. Her classmates called her Pumpkin Frumkin. She dreaded gym class. She was always one of the last two or three girls picked when teams were being formed. When she and a friend named Arlene Epstein, another underdog, whom Sylvia thought to be "different" just as she was, were chosen to complete a team, Sylvia was stung by the other girls' comments: "Ugh, Sylvia — we hit the jackpot," or "Arlene, pugh."

One of the seventh-grade teachers considered Sylvia talented, eager, and friendly; the teacher admired the sensitive poetry she wrote, which was published in the school literary magazine. She noticed that Sylvia was ostracized by most of her contemporaries, and asked one of the popular girls in the class what she and her friends had against Sylvia. The girl told her that Sylvia was uncouth: She picked her nose and scratched herself, and didn't seem aware that such habits were offensive. The teacher began to realize that Sylvia lacked an awareness of how she appeared to others.

Harriet and Irving Frumkin didn't realize that there was anything wrong with Sylvia. To them, her throwing up in the car was simply "a little hyperactivity." In the opinion of some of the Frumkins' friends and relatives, Irving Frumkin saw nothing wrong with Sylvia because he wasn't paying close attention to her. Both Sylvia and Joyce remember that there was constant bickering in the household from the time they were very young. Sylvia remembers hearing her father shout to her mother during one of the family quarrels, "I never wanted a second child!" When Sylvia, the child Irving Frumkin didn't want, failed to measure up to her older sister, he began to ignore her. Sylvia was a lonely girl. When she came home from grade school, her mother was usually giving art lessons, and she was sent to her room and told to be quiet. She resented her mother's students — she often complained that they were her mother's "surrogate children." By then, Joyce was in junior high school and was busy with extracurricular activities. Until Joyce was ten, she had been able to walk to her grandmother's apartment after school, but Minna Wilder had stayed in Brooklyn when the Frumkins moved to Queens, and so Sylvia had had her grandmother's attention and affection only until the age of four. Because Sylvia had few friends and suffered from her father's favoring Joyce, she became close to her mother. She was glad when the day's art lessons were over, so that she and her mother could talk. Harriet Frumkin had resented the way Minna Wilder always favored Benjamin, and was eager to be close to both her daughters. She welcomed Sylvia's confidences. Mrs. Frumkin usually accepted whatever Sylvia told her as true, and took her side against those she claimed had been cruel to her. The first time Sylvia was sorry she had confided in her mother was the summer after she turned fourteen, when a boy at a coed camp she was attending kissed her and fondled her, and then dropped her for another girl. Sylvia enjoyed the young man's fleeting attention, but when she told her mother about the romance her mother got angry and refused to let her go out on dates.

Sylvia graduated from junior high school in June of 1962 with certificates for excellence in several subjects. During ninth grade, she had applied for admission to the High School of Music and Art, in upper Manhattan, one of New York City's best public high schools. One reason she wanted to go to Music and Art was to get away from her junior-high-school classmates, most of whom were going on to the local high school in Queens. Ninth grade had been a particularly unhappy year for Sylvia; she had often come home and told her mother that everyone in the lunchroom was talking about her. Music and Art's students were selected from the city's five boroughs. Sylvia hoped they would be less cliquish. Another reason for going to Music and Art was to surpass Joyce, who hadn't applied there. By 1962, Joyce was experiencing some of the consequences of the pressure her father had put on her. He had convinced her that no matter how well she did, it was never good enough, so she was always unhappy. When she won two prizes at her high school and was twenty-fifth in her class, she felt that she had failed. Her best friend had been second in the class, and two of her friends had won four and seven prizes apiece. She had been an editor of the school newspaper, but not the editor-in-chief; she had been on the cheering squad, but she hadn't been a cheerleader. She told one of several therapists she consulted in later life, "My father always had me competing against an idealized version of Joyce to which I could never measure up."

In September of 1962, the Frumkins felt proud of their daughters. They were pleased that Sylvia was about to start Music and Art, and they had agreed to let her take voice lessons — something she had wanted to do for a long time — as well as art lessons. They were even more pleased that Joyce, who was about to start her senior year in college, had just announced her engagement to Roger Sussman, a first-year medical student at Cornell, whom the Frumkins regarded as a "good catch." Joyce had met Roger at a dance during the fall of her junior year at college. They were going to be married in June of 1963, the Sunday after her graduation. The Frumkins did not suspect that the future would never look so bright to them again.

Twelve

The tenth grade at Music and Art started promisingly for Sylvia. She told her mother that she preferred her new classmates. She complained, however, that she felt under a great deal of strain. The trip from Beechhurst to Music and Art took from an hour and a half to two hours each way. To get to school, Sylvia had to get up at six-thirty and take a bus and two subways. She didn't return home until five o'clock. She had six subjects — English, French, math, biology, world history, and art. The combination of five long school days, a lot of homework, and the Saturday art and voice lessons was too much for her, she said, but she didn't want to give up either the school or the Saturday lessons. That November, Sylvia's friend Arlene, who had gone on to the local public high school, had a nervous breakdown. She spent six weeks at Hillside, a psychiatric hospital in Queens. Arlene's breakdown upset Sylvia. Because she and Arlene had always felt like outcasts, they had become friends of a misery-loves-company kind. They had read books about children who were "different," as they considered themselves to be — children who went to special schools, like Summerhill, in England — and they had gone to see movies about troubled adolescents, such as *Splendor in the Grass.*

While Arlene was at Hillside, Joyce Frumkin decided to break her engagement. She felt that she wasn't good enough for Roger Sussman. Many years later, she told a therapist that when things were going as well for her as they had appeared to be going that fall, they seemed too good to be really happening to imperfect Joyce Frumkin. On a Friday evening in November, she borrowed a college classmate's car for the weekend and drove home to tell her parents that she planned to give Roger his ring back the following week. The Frumkins were horrified. They reminded Joyce that they had already told all their friends about her engagement and her emerald-cut two-carat diamond ring. A broken engagement would cause them great embarrassment, they said, and Joyce might come to regret her decision. They reminded her that in a few years she would be the wife of a prosperous doctor. They persuaded Joyce to proceed with her wedding plans. On Saturday, they went with her to a department store and helped her choose a wedding gown and wedding invitations.

On her way back to college Sunday evening, Joyce drove her classmate's car off the road and into a tree. She received only minor injuries. The car was a total loss. When she called her parents to tell them about the accident, she said she was convinced that it hadn't been an accident. The Frumkins told her that she was being silly; of course it had been an accident, and her friend's insurance company would surely cover it. They said that long-distance telephone calls were expensive. Joyce did not break her engagement.

A few days after the accident, Sylvia told her parents that she was afraid of having a nervous breakdown and winding up at Hillside, like Arlene. She said that she was unhappy and lonely, and that she was sure something was wrong with her. She asked her parents for psychiatric help. It was Sylvia's turn to be told that she was being silly. "No daughter of ours needs psychiatric help," the Frumkins told Sylvia. As one of Joyce's therapists explained to her in 1976, her parents were insecure people who worried a great deal about what others thought of them. Broken engagements and daughters under psychiatric care would reflect badly on them. It was one thing to spend money on art lessons and quite another to spend money on psychiatrists.

Sylvia was determined to be heard. One day in late November, when her parents had been ignoring her requests for psychiatric help for several weeks, she told her mother she was going into the bathroom to cut her wrists. In the bathroom, she touched a razor blade lightly to one wrist. Harriet Frumkin opened the bathroom door, saw a little blood on Sylvia's wrist, and told her that she could go to a woman named Alma Waxman. Mrs. Waxman was a psychiatric social worker with a small private practice in Beechhurst. She had helped the daughter of one of Mrs. Frumkin's friends with some "adolescent problems." Sylvia went to see Mrs. Waxman once a week for three weeks in December. She refused to return for a fourth session, because she didn't like Mrs. Waxman — she wasn't a warm person, Sylvia said. The parting was by mutual consent. Mrs. Waxman called the Frumkins to say that Sylvia was a very troubled fourteen-year-old girl, who needed much more professional help than she could give her. Mrs. Waxman suggested that Sylvia be taken to the Jamaica Center for Psychotherapy — a psychiatric clinic with about seven hundred patients on its rolls, including both children and adults.

On January 24, 1963, Irving Frumkin drove Sylvia to the Jamaica Center, where she was interviewed by the center's chief psychiatric social worker, Gloria Schwartz. This interview was the first step in accepting a prospective patient. After spending an hour and a half with Sylvia, Mrs. Schwartz wrote up a two-page report of the interview. The first subject she covered was "Appearance," and the first line she wrote to describe Sylvia was "She is a tall, unattractive girl." Mrs. Schwartz went on to note Sylvia's untidiness, her restlessness, and her overtalkativeness. She described her affect — her emotional tone — as "shallow" and recorded that she swung readily from tearfulness to giggling. She observed that Sylvia's nails were bitten and her cuticles torn, with "dried blood present around the nails." Moving on to the next heading in her report, "Presenting Problem and History," Mrs. Schwartz wrote that Sylvia felt something was the matter with her because she was overemotional and took things the wrong way. She said that her ninth-grade classmates, who ridiculed her by drawing pictures of her, passing them around, and laughing, were "evil and malicious." She said that although she now had friends who seemed to like her, she believed that they didn't really like her, and she didn't trust them. Sylvia also told Mrs. Schwartz that she had a problem with her parents, who treated her like a child. She said that she was easily angered by them and that when she became angry she yelled, used profane language, cursed, and slapped her father. Sylvia told Mrs. Schwartz that she had been alone and friendless as a child and had had an imaginary friend named Grayson, and that she made up stories about people who were blindfolded, tortured, and kidnapped. At first, she had liked to be the one to kidnap others; now she liked to be the one kidnapped. She enjoyed sex dreams and kidnap dreams. She said she had the feeling that people talked about her, and said she used to hear them doing so; among the things they said was that she ate like a pig. Under "Developmental History and Family Constellation," Mrs. Schwartz put down that Sylvia objected to her mother's nagging. Her father got on her nerves, Sylvia said, because she had the same "bad habits" he had: "He talks loud, monopolizes conversations, interrupts, slurps his soup." The previous summer, Sylvia told Mrs. Schwartz, she had had her first date with a boy, with whom she engaged in petting, and this had left her feeling "unclean and guilty." After she told her parents about this experience, her mother had refused to let her go out on dates. Mrs. Schwartz's "Diagnostic Impression" was that Sylvia Frumkin was suffering from schizophrenia. She arranged for her to be tested by Miriam Abel, a child psychologist, in early February.

On February 9, 1963, Mrs. Abel reported that she had administered four tests to Sylvia Frumkin: an intelligence test (the Wechsler Intelligence Scale for Children, or WISC) and three projective tests — a Rorschach test, a House-Tree-Person test, and the Thematic Apperception Test, or TAT. The subject's associations to inkblots (the Rorschach), the subject's drawings on a blank piece of paper (the House-Tree-Person), and the stories that the subject makes up after viewing stimulus pictures (the TAT) are considered useful diagnostic tools because the material in all three of these tests is so unstructured that any response will reflect some aspect of the subject's underlying personality conflicts and thought processes.

In her report, Mrs. Abel confirmed Sylvia's fears that something was wrong with her. According to Mrs. Abel, an analysis of the projective tests showed that Sylvia was "an extremely anxious, sexually confused girl" who seemed to have a limited ability to control her actions. She was aware of and worried by her fragile controls. "Themes of death, murder, and impending disaster pervade her fantasy life . . . Rape, masturbation, and . . . castration fears are conscious preoccupations." Her intense anger and feelings of frustration were directed toward her parents, whom she thought of as emotionally distant and at times "evil." She felt that both parents rejected her. Mrs. Abel wrote that aggressive and sadomasochistic fantasies were reflected throughout the projective stories, and gave as an example Sylvia's response to a picture of a young boy who was crying: "She stated that a young boy is crying 'because he is upset by what he has done . . . lying next to him is a gun or a knife . . . he just killed his parents.' "

Although there are no tests for schizophrenia comparable to the definitive tests for pregnancy or syphilis, the results of psychological tests may make a diagnosis of schizophrenia more or less probable. The scores of Sylvia Frumkin's WISC test were compatible with a diagnosis of schizophrenia. She had a full-scale IQ of 104, which showed that she was functioning in the average range; a verbal-scale IQ of 113; and a performance-scale IQ of 93. "Verbal facilities are in the bright-normal range, and several of her responses suggest even higher capacities," Mrs. Abel wrote. "By contrast, she had extreme difficulty in handling the performance subtests which required concentration abilities. She obtained a particularly low score on the block-design subtests and resorted to trial-and-error methods. The overall test pattern suggests marked impairment in intellectual functioning due to the emotional difficulties." Mrs. Abel concluded that in view of Sylvia's severe pathology there was an immediate need for treatment. She questioned whether Sylvia could be treated on an out-patient basis. She advised a trial period of therapy with a female therapist, along with medication, but said that hospitalization might become necessary. Mrs. Abel's impression was that Sylvia Frumkin was suffering from a schizophrenic disorder of a paranoid nature. (When Miss Frumkin was given similar projective and intelligence tests three, five, and eleven years later, the results were almost identical.)

The third step in Sylvia's being accepted at the Jamaica Center was an evaluation by Dr. Oliver Cutler, a psychiatrist, on March 8, 1963. Sylvia told Dr. Cutler that when she was young she had had four imaginary friends, and that at present she hallucinated before going to sleep. "She sees two hands trying to thread a needle and failing," Dr. Cutler wrote. "This repeats itself over and over again, and it irritates her. Wishes she was never born. Wishes all her enemies were dead . . . says last year a girl tried to stab her with a compass . . . Wishes to be on her own at times 'with her friend that is inside her.' Feels every man that looks her way is going to attack her." Sylvia admitted to experiencing "occasional trances and momentary auditory hallucinations" when she heard the sound of a motor. Dr. Cutler's diagnosis was paranoid schizophrenia.

⸙ ⸙ ⸙

On March 20, 1963, Sylvia Frumkin started therapy with Dr. Sheila Gross, a child psychiatrist at the Jamaica Center. That afternoon, when she arrived to see Dr. Gross, a middle-aged woman with a European accent, she saw a sheaf of papers on the doctor's desk. The top piece of paper was the first page of Mrs. Schwartz's report. Sylvia made use of her ability to read upside down. She was stunned by the first line on the page — the one that read "She is a tall, unattractive girl." She decided to test Dr. Gross, and asked her to read the page to her. Dr. Gross glanced at Mrs. Schwartz's report, read aloud, "She is a tall girl, not unattractive," and then changed the subject. Although Sylvia went to see Dr. Gross once a week from the end of March to the end of June, she didn't trust her, because the doctor hadn't been honest with her. She felt no rapport with Dr. Gross, because each time she confided something to her Dr. Gross tended to react disapprovingly. When Sylvia told her about her summer romance at camp, Dr. Gross's response was "Ach, you are too young." Despite the fact that Sylvia didn't consider Dr. Gross helpful, she completed tenth grade at Music and Art with an eighty-seven-percent average. No sooner had she done so than Dr. Gross recommended that Sylvia be hospitalized. She was sent to Dr. Donald Greenfeld, a psychiatrist, who was the associate medical director of the Jamaica Center, to be evaluated for hospitalization. Dr. Greenfeld found that Sylvia was adamant about not going to a hospital. He had worked in two state psychiatric hospitals and hadn't thought much of them; he felt that patients were not given much attention in state hospitals. He also believed that he saw sufficient signs of strength in Sylvia Frumkin to keep her on an out-patient basis. Sylvia requested a young female therapist. Dr. Greenfeld assigned her to one, whom she was to start seeing in the fall.

The summer of 1963 was an eventful one for the Frumkins. Joyce graduated in June and was married a few days later. While she was in Europe on her honeymoon and Sylvia was at a camp in Pennsylvania sponsored by a Zionist organization, the Frumkins moved from their apartment in Beechhurst to a pleasant house nearby. Minna Wilder gave the Frumkins the down payment for the house. It had three bedrooms, a bathroom, a dining room, a kitchen, and a living room all on the ground floor, and a finished attic, which Mrs. Frumkin used as a studio and in which she gave her art lessons. By 1963, East New York had deteriorated. Minna Wilder had had an eye operation and could no longer live there safely. Irving Frumkin insisted on giving his mother-in-law the master bedroom of their new house. The Frumkins and Sylvia occupied the two smaller bedrooms.

In September, Sylvia began eleventh grade at Music and Art and began seeing Francine Baden, a young clinical psychologist at the Jamaica Center. At their first session, Sylvia tested Miss Baden as she had tested Sheila Gross — by asking her to read Mrs. Schwartz's report aloud. "She is a tall, unattractive girl," Miss Baden read. Fifteen years later, Miss Frumkin still remembered that first session vividly. "I *was* a tall, unattractive girl," she has said. "The day I went to see Mrs. Schwartz, I was wearing a dirty white blouse over a turtleneck sweater, and a skirt, knee socks, and heels. I told Francine I wasn't dressing well or taking care of myself, and we started talking about why I was making myself unattractive." Miss Frumkin recalled that after they discussed her appearance she started to dress better and to pay more attention to her grooming. She got a stylish haircut and bought some clothes in pink, her favorite color. "I was a pink vision in my new cashmere sheath, pink fishnet stockings, and pink patent-leather shoes," she said one day in the summer of 1978 when she was sitting on the floor of a dayhall in

Creedmoor wearing a dirty orange blouse and a pair of torn red slacks.

One of the other things that Sylvia discussed with Miss Baden was her lack of friends. Early in the eleventh grade, Sylvia had tried to get into a sorority and had been blackballed by two girls. She complained of having too much homework and of having some teachers who were witches. She told Miss Baden she was sorry she hadn't gone to the local high school, where there would have been less pressure. Sylvia also spoke of wanting to go to a special school, like the one depicted in *David and Lisa,* a movie she had seen and loved. She wanted to meet a boy just like David; she wanted to escape her troubles. Miss Baden helped Sylvia realize that Music and Art was an excellent school and that she did have friends, among them the girls who had voted for her to be in the sorority. They talked about some of the things that Sylvia did to make herself unpopular — things like asking other people if they liked her, biting her fingernails, and mumbling — and Sylvia tried to improve her behavior once she realized that it might be irritating to others. She noticed that as soon as she looked better she began to feel better about herself and did make some friends. She was especially fond of a classmate named Camilla Costello, who told her, "Sylvia, I have many friends, but you're my best friend." Sylvia had stopped going to the Saturday sessions at the art school after tenth grade, and had started to enjoy popular music, as many of her new friends did. She bought a number of Beatles records and Paul Anka records; among her favorite songs was Paul Anka's hit tune "Diana." She was behaving more like a typical teen-ager. She started smoking, and she spent hours talking to her friends on the telephone. The more time she spent with her friends, the less time she spent telling her mother her troubles; there were fewer troubles to tell about. She couldn't help noticing that her mother resented her new friends and her good relationship with Miss Baden.

The Frumkins disapproved of most of the changes in their daughter, and blamed Miss Baden for all of them. Mrs. Frumkin preferred classical music to "I Want to Hold Your Hand" and "Diana." Before Sylvia went to see Miss Baden, she had been fairly docile; afterward, she was rebellious. The Jamaica Center charged from ten to fifteen dollars an hour for therapy, depending on the patient's ability to pay. The Frumkins were charged eleven dollars an hour. They wanted to bring in the check themselves. Miss Baden insisted that Sylvia bring it in. She believed it was so important for Sylvia to become an independent person, but so difficult for her to break away from a mother who was unwilling to let go, that she gave her two hours of therapy every week and charged her for only one. Although the sessions were rarely easy and were sometimes painful — Sylvia often tried to evade her problems by chatting about trivia or escaping into fantasy — Miss Baden felt that by January of 1964 they had made some real progress.

⁊ ⁊ ⁊

On the afternoon of Monday, January 27, 1964, Irving Frumkin met Sylvia at the Jamaica Center around six o'clock to drive her home from a session with Miss Baden. He let Sylvia off at a store several blocks from the house, where she bought a package of graph paper for a school project. Mr. Frumkin drove on to a service station to buy some gas. Sylvia walked home from the store. She got as far as the corner directly opposite her house and started to cross the street. When she had almost reached the sidewalk, a car turned the corner at high speed, hit her, threw her fifteen or twenty feet, and hit a lamppost right outside the Frumkins' house. Harriet Frumkin was in the living room and heard a loud crash. She thought that someone might have been hurt, grabbed a coat, and opened the front door. The first thing she saw was the car that had smashed into the lamppost. The second thing she saw was a person lying in the street in front of a neighbor's house. She hurried over and saw that it was her daughter. Sylvia had briefly lost consciousness and was just opening her eyes when her mother reached her. She said that her head ached and so did her legs. Two police cars and an ambulance arrived. By then, Mr. Frumkin had returned home. Mrs. Frumkin rode in the ambulance with Sylvia to the emergency room of nearby Flushing Hospital. Mr. Frumkin followed in his car. The driver who had hit Sylvia — a seventeen-year-old boy — wasn't injured. He was driving alone on a learner's permit — a violation of motor-vehicle regulations. He said he hadn't seen her, because it was dark and she was wearing a black coat.

The doctor who examined Sylvia at Flushing Hospital found a swelling on her head, a swollen and tender left calf, and numerous scrapes and bruises. Subsequent tests and X rays revealed no internal injuries and no broken bones. She was admitted to the hospital and was put to bed with an ice bag on her head and another one on her left calf. She complained of a few aches and pains while she was in Flushing Hospital, but she still recalls her week there with great pleasure. "I remember running around to everyone's room visiting," she said not long ago. "I felt I was on a vacation. It was nice to lie around most of the day and to have my meals served to me in bed." Sylvia was discharged from Flushing Hospital on February 3. Her final diagnosis was multiple contusions and abrasions and a cerebral concussion. She felt well enough to return to Music and Art the day after she got out of the hospital.

Like thousands of other teen-agers in New York City in February of 1964, Miss Frumkin was excited because the Beatles were flying to New York on Friday, February 7, on their first visit to the United States. On Saturday, Sylvia and her friend Camilla Costello went to the Plaza Hotel, where the Beatles were staying, to try to see them. They didn't get into the hotel. Camilla's mother was furious when she learned what the girls had done. The following evening, Sylvia and Camilla went to the studio where the Beatles were going to appear on Ed Sullivan's television show live. Many thousands of teen-age girls wanted to get into the studio. Sylvia and Camilla were among the few hundred who succeeded. After the show, they joined the crowd gathered at the stage door. Mrs. Costello suddenly appeared — she had somehow managed to find out where the girls were. She grabbed Camilla by her coat, pointed at Sylvia, and shouted to her daughter, "You're not to be associated with her anymore!" She then shouted to Sylvia, "And as for you, I hope you have another car accident!" On Thursday, February 13, Sylvia went to LaGuardia Airport to see the Beatles off. Camilla was not with her. That evening, Sylvia called home from the airport. Her father answered the telephone. "I'm at the airport and I'm frightened," Sylvia told him, in a hysterical voice. "I don't know how to get home." Her father said, "How you got there, that's how you get home," and hung up. Sylvia Frumkin got home after midnight; she never told her parents how.

Sylvia had always been nervous and had always done things to excess. Many of her contemporaries had caught Beatlemania, but she had come down with the most virulent case of it. After the car accident, she became increasingly anxious about her schoolwork. She noticed that she would suddenly start giggling for no reason, or suddenly fall silent, or suddenly become hyperactive. She spent more time on the telephone with her friends, she stayed up later doing homework and swallowing No Doz, she smoked three packs of cigarettes a day, she rewrote her school notes, she took several showers a day, she bought and constantly played Beatles records. She told her mother that she was Cinderella, and accused her mother of being her wicked stepmother. Francine Baden was her fairy godmother; her pink patent-leather shoes were her glass slippers; and Paul McCartney was her Prince Charming. She told Miss Baden that she wanted to leave home and live with one of her aunts. In early March, she stayed up all one night figuring out how much money she had in her bank account. She came to several of her sessions with Miss Baden too agitated to talk. The Jamaica Center specialized in psychotherapy, but occasionally its staff psychiatrists prescribed medication as an adjunct to therapy. Dr. Greenfeld had prescribed small doses of Stelazine for Sylvia in 1963 and 1964. Miss Baden stayed late several times when Sylvia was distraught, to give her the medication.

On the morning of Thursday, March 19, 1964, Sylvia Frumkin traveled from Beechhurst to Music and Art, attended her first class of the day, and, when it was over, left the classroom, walked out of the school, and took the subway to the home of her father's youngest brother, Hyman, and his wife, Phyllis. She asked them to adopt her.

Phyllis and Hyman's marriage was an acrimonious one. They fought because Hyman was given to gambling, to flagrant and incessant infidelity, and to shady business deals, and they fought because of Phyllis's fecundity. Hyman enjoyed sleeping with his wife as well as with his many paramours, but he didn't enjoy the consequences of their sexual activity. Phyllis had had two sons, two daughters, and bad luck with birth-control devices; she had had a number of abortions. When she became pregnant again, in 1951, she didn't tell her husband about her latest "accident" until it was too late for another abortion. Hyman remained adamant about not having a fifth child, particularly at that time. His finances fluctuated. Within the family, it was said that "Hyman is always making and losing small fortunes." Whatever he earned, he spent more than he earned. In his pockets Phyllis had found bills for jewelry he had bought for other women when she didn't have enough money in the house to buy groceries. In 1951, Hyman was in debt. He had borrowed several thousand dollars from a few of his relatives, including Phyllis's brother Ralph Stadtman. "This time, either the crib goes or I go," he told his wife, and she called her sister-in-law Harriet to report her husband's reaction to the news of the prospective arrival of their fifth child. It was one of many lines that became part of the family folklore, and was often repeated to Sylvia and Joyce. Ralph Stadtman and his wife, Donna, were childless, though they had been trying for years to have a baby. Several months before Hyman and Phyllis Frumkin's baby was due, they arranged to let Ralph and Donna adopt it. The Stadtmans agreed to pay Phyllis's hospital bills and to forget about the money that Hyman owed them. After the birth of the baby — a girl, whom the Stadtmans named Ruth — they took her home from the hospital and moved to Philadelphia. It was beyond the Irving Frumkins' understanding that anyone could part with a child. "Even gypsies stole children; they didn't sell them," Harriet Frumkin often observed. Nevertheless, the two couples remained friendly, perhaps because the Irving Frumkins were fascinated by a way of living that was the opposite of their own. Harriet and Irving Frumkin were frugal people, who always lived well within their means. If they had two thousand dollars to spend on a car, they bought a Chevrolet for eighteen hundred dollars and put two hundred dollars in the bank. For many years after the advent of television, their only television set was a small black-and-white model. Hyman and Phyllis were enthusiastic practitioners of conspicuous consumption. If they had two thousand dollars, they used the money as a down payment on a Cadillac and took out a loan for the balance. The Hyman Frumkins were the first people the Irving Frumkins knew to buy a color-television set. In the late 1950s, Hyman Frumkin went into the business of manufacturing stereo equipment. In the early sixties, when stereo equipment became increasingly popular, Hyman Frumkin made another small fortune, and bought a large house in Jamaica Estates, Queens. He and Phyllis furnished it with crushed-velvet sofas, sculptured wall-to-wall carpeting, and lamps whose bases were nude women. Sylvia was especially taken with Hyman and Phyllis. When she was fifteen, she thought that they were "finer" people than her parents, simply because they were richer.

The Hyman Frumkins' wealth wasn't the only reason that Sylvia went to their home on the morning of March 19 and asked them to adopt her. She also went there because she could no longer stand living at home. She thought that she could get along better with Phyllis, who had always been warm toward her, than with her own mother. Still another reason was that she had recently started to fantasize that she wasn't her parents' daughter. She had come to believe that she was really Hyman and Phyllis's child — the one they had sold. Hyman and Phyllis were both home with colds on March 19 when Sylvia rang their doorbell. They were startled to see her, and more startled when she asked them to adopt her. They suggested that she return at once to Music and Art. She told them she didn't need school anymore. When they suggested that she might have a fever and should go home and rest, she became overwrought. She insisted that she was no longer Sylvia Frumkin — that her name was Linette. She started to cry, and then she started to dance around the living room. Phyllis didn't know what to do with her niece. She called Harriet Frumkin to tell her that Sylvia was at their house and was behaving very strangely. Mrs. Frumkin told Phyllis to tell Sylvia to go directly to the Jamaica Center and wait for her on the corner outside, where she would meet her. Mrs. Frumkin called her husband at the bottling company; he said he was busy. Mrs. Frumkin then called Joyce, who had divorced Roger Sussman six months after their marriage. Joyce Frumkin (she had taken back her maiden name) had a job as an apprentice fashion coordinator in Manhattan's garment district and was living in a studio apartment in Greenwich Village. She arranged to leave work, and drove to the Jamaica Center and met her mother and Sylvia. Harriet, Joyce, and Sylvia Frumkin went into the Jamaica Center and talked to Dr. Greenfeld. After Dr. Greenfeld had observed Sylvia and pieced together an account of her behavior that morning and over the past several days, he decided that she had had a psychotic break and required immediate hospitalization. He telephoned Gracie

Square, a hospital on Manhattan's Upper East Side, and arranged for her to be admitted. Dr. Greenfeld thought that Sylvia would get over her acute psychotic episode in a few days.

A week later, Francine Baden wrote up a summary report of Sylvia Frumkin's six months in therapy. It read, in part:

> Sylvia was seen at the Jamaica Center for Psychotherapy twice weekly (one session was free) since September 1963. At first, she was quite resistive, and it was apparent that there was an intense investment in remaining disturbed, miserable, and poorly functioning. One, it provided her with a sense of individuality, as she felt behaving more appropriately meant "conforming." Two, she obtained attention in this highly masochistic way. Three, there was (and is) an intense symbiotic relationship with her mother. Her mother was critical of the therapist for Sylvia, and told Sylvia that the latter was no good and was not helping her. Therefore, if Sylvia did not improve, this meant her mother was right about the therapist and she was thus pleasing her mother. Four, Sylvia's "crying out her problems" about her unpopularity and misery called forth the sympathy, comfort, and overprotective attention from her mother (which was not forthcoming if Sylvia functioned adequately) . . .
>
> It is felt that the case problem is the symbiotic tie with her mother, from which she is now struggling to free herself, and the mutual rage between the mother and herself. She used to tell her mother every event, thought, fantasy, etc. of her life, and felt intensely guilty if she kept any detail from her mother or didn't tell her the truth. She was strongly supported in therapy in this regard — that she had a right to be a separate person, have privacy, and be different from her mother. Sylvia began to be aware that if she was functioning reasonably well, and was not crying on her mother's shoulder, that her mother became resentful and rejecting. As she needed her parents less, her rage exploded into consciousness, and she became terrified of her own impulses to kill them or herself, and hence her violent need to separate herself from them.
>
> A few days before her psychotic break, Sylvia revealed that when she saw her mother screaming and nagging her for

sympathy because she wasn't feeling well, Sylvia felt intensely disgusted and afraid that she would grow up like that. She also said bitterly, "No wonder I didn't have friends, if I was like that."

Despite the pathology, it is felt that this youngster has real strengths, and is fighting to integrate herself, and to be well and happy, and to separate herself from her family (although there is enormous conflict, anxiety and guilt about it). She is unusually bright, talented, sensitive, and has rich potentialities. It is felt that a very warm, strong and positive relationship has been established with the therapist.

She needs to establish her individuality and identity as a separate person through constructive and healthy means, and to identify with a woman and work out the intense rage toward her parents.

In conclusion, Miss Baden wrote, "Considering the extensive pathology of this family, particularly the fantastic pressure of the mother, her profound rejection and hostility of Sylvia, her clutching demandingness and hysterical reactions, it speaks for Sylvia's strengths that she is so desperately trying to pull away. She has excellent insight and is strongly motivated to get well. It is felt that she can make significant gains and progress with psychotherapy."

⸙ ⸙ ⸙

The doctor who admitted Sylvia Frumkin to Gracie Square Hospital on the afternoon of March 19, on a minor voluntary application (at the age of fifteen, she was too young to sign herself into a psychiatric hospital), found her alternately very angry and behaving in a silly and inappropriate manner. One of her prominent symptoms, which she was to display during most of her hospital admissions over the next seventeen years, was marked pressure of speech. She expressed her fear of being judged irrational by saying repeatedly, "Thank God, I still know what's going on." She didn't admit to any hallucinations. The doctor prescribed 200 milligrams of Thorazine per day for her — a reasonable starting dose. Two days later, when she failed to show any improvement, the doctor raised her medication to 800 milligrams of Thorazine per day — a moderate dose. The following day, he gave her 5 milligrams of Stelazine in addition to Thorazine, along with Cogentin, an anti-parkinsonian drug, to keep her from developing the tremors and rigidity that drugs like Thorazine and Stelazine were known to cause. Sylvia Frumkin continued to talk like a baby and to babble excitedly, so her medication was again increased. On March 23, when she received 16 milligrams of Stelazine and 1200 milligrams of Thorazine, she began to show a gradual lessening of the pressure and more control over her thinking. It soon became obvious, however, that she would need more than a week or ten days in a hospital, which was what Dr. Greenfeld had originally anticipated. Gracie Square was a private psychiatric hospital, and Mr. Frumkin's Blue Cross/Blue Shield benefits could not be used to pay the cost of Sylvia's semiprivate room there, which came to thirty-five dollars a day. Dr. Greenfeld helped the Frumkins make arrangements for Sylvia to be transferred to St. Vincent's. St. Vincent's, the largest Catholic hospital on the East Coast, was a general hospital that had a separate mental-health pavilion, where patients were covered by Blue Cross/Blue Shield for periods of up to ninety days. On April 2, 1964, Joyce Frumkin drove Sylvia and her mother from Gracie Square Hospital to the Jacob Reiss Mental Health Pavilion of St. Vincent's, in Greenwich Village. The final diagnosis of the doctor at Gracie Square was that Miss Frumkin was afflicted with acute undifferentiated schizophrenia. He evaluated her condition as improved, her prognosis as fair. Throughout Sylvia's stay at Gracie Square, she had talked jabberwocky about the Beatles. On the drive to St. Vincent's, she insisted that Paul McCartney was going to come and take her away to England.

⁊ ⁊ ⁊

Sylvia Frumkin struck the psychiatric resident who admitted her to St. Vincent's as an appealing but slovenly young girl who was completely overwhelmed by her symptoms. She was exceedingly hyperactive and was in a state of panic. Her thoughts, though quite disconnected, displayed an intellectual orientation to reality but were almost completely dissociated from her affect, which was "blunt." (A blunt affect — meaning there was no visible display of emotions — was another symptom that was frequently observed on Miss Frumkin's many hospital admissions.) She was immediately placed on a daily dosage of 2000 milligrams of Thorazine. She also received some Stelazine at St. Vincent's, and a prophylactic dose of Artane, another anti-parkinsonian drug, similar to Cogentin.

Miss Frumkin remembers that the nurses at St. Vincent's, some of whom were nuns, took very good care of her and that she was fond of one of the occupational therapists, but that she couldn't participate in much occupational therapy, because she was too sick. She kept having delusions that she was The Patient and that all the other eighty-five patients at St. Vincent's were reflections of her personality whose presence was required so that she could learn to live with herself. Her only really happy memory of St. Vincent's is of receiving a ten-page letter written on lined yellow legal-size paper from her friend Camilla Costello. Harriet Frumkin has no pleasant memories of St. Vincent's. She recalls that Sylvia was extremely hostile and that most of her hostility was directed at her mother. On May 5, 1964, Sylvia's sixteenth birthday, Mrs. Frumkin brought her a birthday cake. Sylvia refused to open the cake box and shoved it back at her mother, saying, "You got me in here, now you get out of here and take your rotten cake with you." The hospital staff asked Mrs. Frumkin to leave, and not to return until they called her, because of the upsetting effect she had on her daughter. Mrs. Frumkin departed in tears. "Whenever Sylvia is sick, she's especially nasty to me, because I gave birth to her," Mrs. Frumkin said recently. "If it hadn't been for me, she wouldn't have been born, so she wouldn't have been sick." The resident at St. Vincent's did not permit Francine Baden to visit, either, when Sylvia asked to see her; he told Sylvia that she was supposed to relate only to him, and not to her previous therapist.

Within a few weeks, the resident observed an improvement in Sylvia's condition. Once she appeared "more organized and able to sustain some attention and direction for short periods," he gradually lowered her daily medication from 2000 milligrams of Thorazine to 400 milligrams. For reasons that he described simply as "obscure," her condition then took a sudden turn for the worse. On June 19, she claimed that she had swallowed a piece of wood with loosely attached nails. No one had witnessed this act. A nurse removed a piece of wood and a nail from her mouth. X rays were taken immediately. No radio-opaque foreign bodies were identified in the gastrointestinal tract. The wood-and-nails incident was regarded by the hospital staff as an attention-getting device. A few hours later, Sylvia swallowed almost an entire bottle of shampoo — an act that the staff regarded as a more serious suicidal gesture. The reasons for the deterioration in Sylvia Frumkin's condition did not seem at all "obscure" to a specialist in psychopharmacology who recently reviewed her record. A slight increase in her attention span was not a sufficient improvement in her condition to justify a major reduction in her medication, he said. He observed that the resident at St. Vincent's would probably have helped her more by raising her dose of Thorazine until her symptoms were well in remission, and only then beginning to lower it gradually to a maintenance dose — which is often about one-third of the peak dose.

Thirteen

When Thorazine, Stelazine, Mellaril, Compazine, and Trilafon — all of them members of a group of drugs called the phenothiazines — were first used in the United States, in the 1950s, they were called tranquilizers. Later, as Miltown and, still later, Librium and Valium came to be widely employed and generally referred to as tranquilizers, psychiatrists began to distinguish between these two distinctive groups of drugs by calling the former major tranquilizers and the latter minor tranquilizers. They soon regretted this nomenclature by comparison, because it gave the false impression that these drugs were of the same type, with one group simply stronger than the other. The minor tranquilizers are completely ineffective in treating the symptoms of psychosis, and are all potentially addictive. What the minor tranquilizers have in common with the major tranquilizers is that both have anti-anxiety effects; the minor tranquilizers are now more accurately called anti-anxiety drugs. The major tranquilizers — which are not addictive — were eventually renamed antipsychotic drugs, not only in an attempt to differentiate them from the minor tranquilizers but also to clear up a common misconception that they worked by making people groggy and easily manageable. Unlike the barbiturates that were used in mental hospitals for decades, these drugs don't work by putting people to sleep or dulling their senses. They work by reducing the hallucinations, the delusions, and the thinking disorders characteristic of the psychotic phase of schizophrenia and other psychoses, without putting psychotic patients to sleep. More recently, many psychopharmacologists have preferred to call these drugs neuroleptics, for they are all capable of producing certain neurological side effects. In addition, some neuroleptics were found to be useful in other branches of medicine. Compazine, for example, is useful for treating nausea and vomiting, and a parent is more likely to give it to a normal child if it is called a neuroleptic than if it is called an antipsychotic. Twenty neuroleptics are currently in use in the United States; many others are used in other parts of the world.

For some years after Thorazine and the other neuroleptics were introduced, it was not known how they worked. In the last few years, psychopharmacologists have achieved a better understanding of this. There are hundreds of billions of cells in the brain called neurons, which interconnect. The connecting points between neurons are called synapses. At most synapses, a chemical known as a neurotransmitter is released at the end of one neuron, travels a minute distance to the next neuron, and influences that neuron to transmit the impulse. About a score of different neurotransmitters are known today, and a large number are probably yet to be discovered. The neurotransmitter that has been most implicated in schizophrenia is dopamine. During the psychotic phase of schizophrenia, there seems to be an excess of dopamine transmission in the neurons in specific areas of the brain. All the neuroleptics are known to block the dopamine receptors so that the dopamine released at the end of one neuron cannot get to the receptor site of the next neuron.

More than ninety percent of all schizophrenic patients undergoing their first psychotic episode will respond to any one of the twenty neuroleptics if the proper dose is given for the proper length of time. One neuroleptic is thus normally no more effective than another in ridding a patient of delusions, despite claims of drug companies to the contrary. The drugs do, however, have different side effects. The reason that a knowledgeable doctor usually prescribes one neuroleptic rather than another for a patient with no prior history of treatment is that he is familiar with a drug or knows that it has a particular spectrum of side effects. Thorazine is one of the neuroleptics that have a strong sedative side effect. A number of specialists in psychopharmacology have gone so far as to call it "obsolete" and have ceased to use it clinically, because it has numerous undesirable side effects, including the oversedation. The sedative property is the characteristic that makes it especially popular in understaffed state hospitals, where attendants find heavily sedated patients easier to control. Thorazine is one of the most commonly prescribed drugs at Creedmoor.

In the mid-sixties, Thorazine and Stelazine, which are manufactured by the same drug company, were often given simultaneously, as they were to Sylvia Frumkin at Gracie Square and at St. Vincent's in 1964. The theory behind giving patients both Thorazine and Stelazine was that the patients would get the combined therapeutic effects of both drugs, and that the side effects would be fewer or would cancel each other out. This combination of two neuroleptics was approved by the Food and Drug Administration on the basis of inadequate scientific evidence. Subsequent evidence showed clearly that there was rarely any advantage in prescribing Thorazine and Stelazine simultaneously, but that there was a disadvantage, because patients got the full side effects of both drugs: sedation, dryness of mouth, lowering of blood pressure, and tremors. Another unfortunate consequence of the FDA's approval of this combination (which many psychiatrists still prescribe frequently) is that it gave the agency's blessing to polypharmacy — the administering of simultaneous doses of two, three, four, or more neuroleptics. For the schizophrenic patients on whom a particular neuroleptic is ineffective, a knowledgeable psychiatrist will switch from that neuroleptic to another that has a different molecular structure. To facilitate the switching, most psychiatrists have access to an equivalency table. Equivalency tables are based on 100 milligrams of Thorazine and show the amount of one drug that is approximately equal to the amount of another. For example, Mellaril and Serentil are two neuroleptics of low-milligram potency, like Thorazine: A hundred milligrams of Mellaril is the equivalent of 100 milligrams of Thorazine, and 50 milligrams of Serentil is the equivalent of 100 milligrams of Thorazine. Most neuroleptics are high-milligram-potency drugs; thus, 10 milligrams of Trilafon or Moban is the equivalent of 100 milligrams of Thorazine.

The resident at St. Vincent's who prematurely lowered Miss Frumkin's dose of Thorazine was committing an error that illustrates the difficulty of prescribing neuroleptics. In many fields of medicine, it is relatively easy to prescribe drugs, because there are standard doses for whole classes of ailments, and these can be memorized. For the infectious diseases that are responsive to the tetracycline antibiotics, for instance, the adult dosage is usually 250 milligrams four times a day; in some cases, the dose is twice that. There are no standard doses in psychiatry. For one patient, 200 milligrams of Thorazine may be sufficient to clear up the delusions over a period of time; another may require 2000 milligrams to achieve the same result. Studies have been done which demonstrate that if you give a group of patients a standard dose of a certain tricyclic antidepressant (a chemical class of antidepressants characterized by a three-ringed molecular structure), and then, after a sufficient period of time, measure the level of the drug in the blood, one individual may have as much as a hundred times the amount that another has. Other less dramatic but still significant differences are quite common. The drug levels in the blood of identical twins are almost identical; those of close relatives show a high correlation; those of strangers show no correlation. Currently, it is routine to measure blood levels of lithium, and in the past several years it has become possible to measure the blood levels of tricyclic antidepressants in clinical psychiatric practice, as distinct from a research setting. These measurements can provide psychiatrists with a better guide to prescribing adequate doses of such drugs. Only recently has it become possible to measure the blood levels of neuroleptics, but the clinical value of these measurements has not yet been conclusively determined. For the seventeen years that Sylvia Frumkin has been on neuroleptics, therefore, psychiatrists have been prescribing drugs for her simply on the basis of her observed responses. Many fifteen-year-olds suffering their first psychotic breaks respond to 500 milligrams of Thorazine within ten days. Sylvia Frumkin's failure to respond quickly or favorably to much higher doses of Thorazine indicated a poorer prognosis for treatment.

⁄ ⁄ ⁄

In 1964, voluntary hospitals like St. Vincent's wanted "good" patients, not troublesome ones. Shortly after Sylvia Frumkin swallowed shampoo, her parents were told that because she had "regressed to her pre-admission state of disorganization," St. Vincent's would be able to do nothing further to help her during the ten or twelve days that remained before the ninety-day period covered by Irving Frumkin's insurance expired. The resident said that Sylvia would need long-term hospital care. For everyone but a few of the very rich who are able both to afford private hospitals and to find the private hospitals willing to accept difficult cases, this means going to a state hospital. In 1964 (as in 1981), the state hospital that served the residents of Queens was Creedmoor. Patients at Creedmoor were billed seven dollars a day in 1964. When Sylvia Frumkin was discharged, the St. Vincent's resident diagnosed her illness as acute schizophrenia, undifferentiated, unimproved.

In 1964, the only way a patient in a hospital like St. Vincent's could be admitted to a state hospital was by way of a city hospital, such as Bellevue. On June 22, 1964, therefore, Sylvia was taken by ambulance from St. Vincent's to Bellevue. Mrs. Frumkin, Joyce, and an attendant from St. Vincent's accompanied her on the short ride. Sylvia was fairly calm in the ambulance, although she was troubled by the idea of being transferred to yet another hospital. "Is there no place on earth for me?" she asked her mother in a plaintive voice. It was a question that Sylvia asked her mother dozens of times over the next seventeen years. Her admission to Bellevue was merely a paper admission, but it took a while. Sylvia became wilder as time dragged on. After three hours, she was admitted to an ambulance bound for Creedmoor instead of to a ward at Bellevue. In the ambulance there were several other patients and a policeman. With its back window protected by wire mesh, and with long, hard benches inside, the ambulance resembled a paddy wagon. Joyce and Mrs. Frumkin followed the ambulance out to Creedmoor in Joyce's car.

As soon as Mrs. Frumkin saw Building 40, Creedmoor's seventeen-story skyscraper, from the Grand Central Parkway, she thought back sadly to 1962, when she and her husband had felt so proud of their daughters, with Joyce having just announced her engagement and with Sylvia about to start at Music and Art. Mrs. Frumkin had heard of Creedmoor in 1962, but she had never seen the hospital, let alone imagined that one of her daughters would wind up there. "Creedmoor" was then just a word that a friend might use in a sentence like "He's so crazy he should be in Creedmoor." By the time Mrs. Frumkin and Joyce reached Creedmoor, where Mr. Frumkin met them, they were emotionally drained. Sylvia was in a rage. Building 40, which had opened in 1960, was then Creedmoor's newest building. It served as the hospital's medical building and contained its admissions wards. Patients who improved quickly were discharged from Building 40. Those who didn't were dispatched, after a period of twelve to eighteen months, to the "back wards," which were located in a large number of three- and four-story buildings that were spread out on Creedmoor's three-hundred-acre site.

Sylvia Frumkin was admitted to Creedmoor by Dr. Ida Feller, a psychiatrist on the women's-reception staff. Sylvia was very upset that her father had to sign the forms required to admit her on a voluntary application for a minor, and claimed that she was "a grown-up lady." The Frumkins gave Dr. Feller, a European-born woman in her fifties, a synopsis of the recent events in Sylvia's life: her schooling, her therapy at the Jamaica Center, her car accident, her fifteen days at Gracie Square, and her eighty-two days at St. Vincent's, including her attempt to drink a bottle of shampoo. Sylvia told Dr. Feller that "Sylvia died in the accident." She also said that she invented new names for herself and imagined she was somebody else. She told the psychiatrist she had run away to her aunt and uncle and wanted them to adopt her, because she couldn't get along with her parents. Dr. Feller's diagnosis was schizophrenia, undifferentiated type. Sylvia was put in Ward 10-A, the women's new-admissions ward, and was started on a daily dose of 300 milligrams of Thorazine — an even smaller dose than the one that had been insufficient to alleviate her symptoms at St. Vincent's.

On June 26, four days after her arrival, a doctor assigned to 10-A interviewed Sylvia Frumkin and wrote up a mental-status report. His principal findings were that she was very agitated, that her thoughts were dissociated, and that she expressed suicidal intention, paranoid ideation, and delusions of persecution. Her affect was "flat," her mood was hostile, and her insight and judgment were impaired. In his report, the doctor included a sample of the dialogue he had exchanged with her:

> I want to go to Freedomland with Paul Anka. (Do you know him?) No, but he knows me. I've lost the feeling that I'm Diana the Goddess. I have to face reality. Maybe I'm not Diana. I don't know. (Hear voices?) I talk to Paul. I hear his voice all the time. (People against you?) Yes — No I don't know. (Feel like committing suicide?) Yes, plenty of times. (Have you tried?) Yes. All kinds of things, razor blades, cigarettes. (Anything else?) I don't remember. I don't want to be normal. Are you going to tear down everything? I want to be Diana — I'm not sick. I want to be Diana. That's all I want to be. I had a crackup three months ago. I don't really consider myself sick, though. I want to run in the wind. No, not really.

Although the attendants in Ward 10-A wrote in their progress notes that Miss Frumkin was restless, nervous, and confused, her daily dose of Thorazine was lowered to 200 milligrams on July 16. The specialist in psychopharmacology who recently reviewed her record said that lowering the dose instead of raising it could be described only as "irrational and incompetent." Three or four hundred milligrams of Thorazine might have been a reasonable starting dose, but when it was ineffective the only sensible thing to do was to raise the dose. He pointed out that in the mid-sixties Creedmoor was noted for undermedicating its patients.

Although Ward 10-A at Creedmoor was not as attractive as Gracie Square or St. Vincent's, it was one of the most pleasant wards at Creedmoor in 1964. It contained the new, and thus usually the most promising, patients, some of the hospital's most modern furniture, and a high ratio of staff to patients. When Sylvia Frumkin became unruly in mid-July and mid-August — she snatched food from other patients, fought with them, refused to wear shoes, and ran up and down the hallway — she was sent from Ward 10-A to Ward 11-A, one of Building 40's "overactive" wards, for aggressive and assaultive women patients. It was then, Mrs. Frumkin remembers, that the real horror of Sylvia's hospitalization hit her. Many of the patients in 11-A were kept in straitjackets, the ward was noisy, and there were few organized activities. On August 12, Sylvia was taking 200 milligrams a day of Thorazine and 4 milligrams a day of Stelazine — the equivalent altogether of 280 milligrams of Thorazine. That day, a psychiatrist wrote on her chart, "Patient did not show much improvement on drug therapy . . . and, therefore, she will start a series of ECT today."

Electroconvulsive therapy, or ECT, commonly called electroshock, had been introduced in New York State psychiatric hospitals in the early 1940s. Before the advent of Thorazine, in 1954, the frequency with which ECT was given increased each year. After Thorazine, the use of ECT declined precipitously. In 1964, Sylvia Frumkin was among the one percent of the patients at Creedmoor who received ECT. Between August 12 and September 4, Miss Frumkin was given eleven shock treatments — one every two or three days. After the first two treatments, attendants noted an improvement in her condition; they described her in their notes as "pleasant, talkative, cooperative." On August 23, after five treatments, she was given grounds privileges. After she had completed eleven treatments, she was able to make weekend visits to her parents' home or to Joyce's apartment. The Frumkins described Sylvia's improvement on ECT as "nothing short of a miracle." Sylvia has only vague memories — none of them painful or traumatic — of the ECT treatments she received at Creedmoor in 1964 and of subsequent ECT treatments she received at Creedmoor and at several other hospitals. The specialist in psychopharmacology who reviewed her record was not impressed by the "miracle" of ECT. "We know in 1981 and we knew in 1964 that ECT is not the treatment of choice for schizophrenic patients with her symptoms," he said. "I think she should have been given adequate medication. There are two possible explanations for her sudden improvement in 1964. Most likely, the ECT worked. It occasionally does work the first few times it's used on some schizophrenics, despite being generally inappropriate. ECT is still the preferred method of treatment for some severe forms of depression and catatonic schizophrenia. There's also the possibility that, coincidentally, her first acute episode of schizophrenia was already coming to an end. Schizophrenia is often an episodic illness. Even in the old days, when hospitals had no drugs and no shock therapy, it often took several episodes of schizophrenia before the patient who returned to the state hospital never got out again."

In September of 1964, plans were being made for Sylvia's discharge from Creedmoor. The Frumkins had sued the young man who hit their daughter with his car on January 27 and the young man's father, the owner of the car. Because the lawsuit was pending that fall, Sylvia's case was presented as "a case of interest" at a general staff meeting — a weekly gathering of administrators, doctors, and residents — on September 25. By then, Mrs. Frumkin was attributing Sylvia's illness to the car accident, and she continued to do so for the next seventeen years. "When she opened her eyes after she was hit, they were never the same," Mrs. Frumkin says.

The psychiatric profession has never agreed on the causes of schizophrenia or other mental illnesses. The disagreement is sometimes referred to, with alliterative simplicity, as "nature versus nurture." The controversy is more complicated than that. It arises out of the conflict between the Platonic concept that the mind and the body are separate and independent entities — a concept that was unchallenged in Western thought until relatively recently — and the concept, derived from modern science, that the mind and the body are one, the mind being just a manifestation of the workings of the brain. The side of the controversy that Francine Baden represents — the so-called nurture school — harks back to the Platonic concept. The theory of this school of psychiatrists and psychologists is that mental illness is wholly a troubling of the mind caused by a poor environment — that is, poor human relationships, which invariably date back to childhood. While Miss Baden did not use the term *schizophrenogenic mother* — schizophrenia-causing mother — she singled out the figure most often blamed by this school for a child's improper nurture: the mother. "It is felt that the case problem is the symbiotic tie with her mother," Miss Baden had written in her summary report on Sylvia Frumkin. She had concluded her statement by proposing the treatment method advocated by this school — psychotherapy. The theory holds that since the illness is caused by faulty human relationships, it can be successfully treated by appropriate psychological intervention to change the relationships and the patient's pattern of behavior and thought.

The opposing side in the controversy, the so-called nature school, consists of biologically oriented psychiatrists, who have followed to its logical conclusion the concept of the mind developed by modern science. Their theory holds that mental illness is a physiological or biochemical imbalance in the body that is affecting the brain, and should be treated with physical remedies. Ironically, Sigmund Freud lent some support to the thinking of this school. He believed that psychoanalysis could do little for schizophrenics and other psychotics, as opposed to neurotics, and that drugs might have a significant impact on psychiatry. "The future may teach us how to exercise a direct influence by particular chemical substances," he predicted. Early adherents of this school pointed to two physical ailments accompanied by psychotic symptoms — pellagra, a vitamin-deficiency disease, which is treated by administering niacinamide to the patient in order to supply him with niacin; and general paresis, a late stage of syphilis that affects the brain and was treated originally with arsenicals and subsequently with penicillin — as evidence that their theory was tenable. These biologically oriented psychiatrists were the practitioners who prescribed sedative packs and continuous-flow tubs in the 1920s, insulin-coma therapy and electroshock therapy in the 1930s and 1940s, and, starting in the 1950s, the antipsychotic drugs. They had also long suspected that heredity was a factor in mental illness. By the early 1970s, enough research had been done to strongly suggest that — at least for a number of serious mental illnesses, including schizophrenia — the biologically oriented psychiatrists were right about both chemical imbalances and genetic factors.

Eugen Bleuler, a Swiss psychiatrist, whose book *Dementia Praecox; or, The Group of Schizophrenias* was published in 1911, coined the word *schizophrenia,* but used it in the plural. The third, and latest, edition of the American Psychiatric Association's *Diagnostic and Statistical Manual of Mental Disorders,* which was published in 1980, uses *schizophrenia* in the singular but says in a footnote that it is to be considered in the plural. The most enlightened current thinking is that schizophrenia is a variety of illnesses, many of which clearly have a genetic factor that has not yet been entirely documented. (There may also be some rare forms of schizophrenia that have other causes.) In this century, the incidence of schizophrenia in all societies where statistics have been kept and analyzed — in the United States and in countries in Africa, Asia, and Europe — is in the neighborhood of one percent. Studies show that the likelihood that a child with one schizophrenic parent will be schizophrenic is ten percent. If both parents are schizophrenics, the odds are at least thirty percent. The genetics of schizophrenia do not appear to be simple. According to one widely held genetic theory, the genetic disposition can be so powerful that the individual will manifest schizophrenic symptoms no matter how benevolent the environment in which he or she is raised. The environmental factor becomes more important when the individual inherits a moderate or low predisposition to schizophrenia. If the environment is a good one, there is a fair chance that a person with a moderate predisposition to schizophrenia will not manifest its symptoms. If there is a low genetic predisposition to schizophrenia and the environment is good, the chances are even less. An individual with a low disposition to schizophrenia who went into the army might be able to go through basic training and combat — two forms of high stress — without manifesting schizophrenia, but if he should be taken prisoner and subjected to harsh conditions, such as brainwashing, these conditions might trigger the illness. A person who is without genes for schizophrenia might emerge from a POW camp with severe neurotic, psychosomatic, or depressive symptoms, but no amount of stress could make him a schizophrenic.

When Sylvia Frumkin was hospitalized at Gracie Square in 1964, her parents were asked if there had been any mental illness in the family. They replied that there hadn't. The doctor taking the record wrote, "Family history reveals no neuropsychiatric disease." Like many families in a similar situation, the Frumkins had not been candid with the doctor. Irving Frumkin's brother Julius had to be put in a psychiatric hospital twice during his late teens. Afterward, he was unable to go to college as the family had hoped he would. He was able to hold a series of menial jobs, the longest-lasting of them as a deliveryman for a florist. He always lived at home — with both parents until his father's death, in 1954; with his mother until her death, in 1972; and then alone, in the same apartment, until his own death, in 1977. Sylvia and Joyce Frumkin remember that when they visited their paternal grandparents Uncle Julius never spoke to them. One day, Sylvia asked him a question about a book he was reading. He walked out of the room and slammed the door in her face. Irving Frumkin does not like to admit that there was anything irregular about his family, but when he is pressed to do so he will acknowledge that his brother Julius was a schizophrenic. It was not until 1979 that his wife learned that his parents had been first cousins; for over forty years, he had allowed her to assume that they were third or fourth cousins. When psychiatrists have asked Harriet

Frumkin if there was any mental illness on her side of the family, she has never told them that her Aunt Vera spent the last years of her life in Pilgrim State Hospital. As well as can be determined, Sylvia Frumkin probably inherited at least a moderate genetic predisposition to schizophrenia, and her childhood environment was sufficiently stressful to trigger the illness. In early 1963, when she was fourteen — roughly a year before the automobile accident and her hospitalization at Gracie Square — a psychiatric social worker, a psychologist, and a psychiatrist at the Jamaica Center for Psychotherapy had successively diagnosed her as a schizophrenic.

After the psychiatrists who considered Sylvia Frumkin's case at the general staff meeting at Creedmoor on September 25, 1964, interviewed her about her psychiatric history, it was their unanimous opinion that her mental illness had begun before the car accident. Unfortunately for the Frumkins, the lawyers for the driver's insurance company subpoenaed the records. The Frumkins were subsequently able to obtain from the director of Creedmoor a statement that "Miss Frumkin's mental status may have been aggravated by the accident in which she was involved," and they were able to get two psychiatrists to testify in court to the same effect. In the spring of 1971, the case was finally settled, for twenty thousand dollars. Shortly after the general staff meeting, Sylvia Frumkin was recommended for discharge. She was advised to take a hundred milligrams of Thorazine daily after her discharge, as a maintenance dosage, and to seek private psychiatric care.

Fourteen

Over the years of Sylvia Frumkin's illness, Harriet Frumkin has judged the psychiatrists who have treated her daughter on the basis of two criteria: how well Sylvia did while she was in their care, and how friendly and optimistic they were. Mrs. Frumkin had disliked the psychiatric resident at St. Vincent's not only because Sylvia's condition hadn't improved there but also because he had seemed cool and foreboding. "Don't be fooled by Sylvia's seeming wellness," he had warned Mrs. Frumkin. "The veneer is very thin." The Frumkins had liked Dr. Feller, who admitted Sylvia to Creedmoor. She had appeared to be concerned about Sylvia. "She is young and intelligent, and she has her whole life ahead of her," Dr. Feller had told them. In early October, when the Frumkins were informed that their daughter should continue in private therapy after her discharge, they chose Dr. Feller as Sylvia's future therapist and sought her help in making plans for Sylvia's education. Sylvia, Harriet and Irving Frumkin, and Dr. Feller agreed that it would be unwise for Sylvia to return to Music and Art. The strain of commuting there had been too great. Besides, Sylvia didn't want to return, because she had completed only half of the eleventh grade and she would have to repeat the year while her former classmates were in twelfth grade. She longed to go to Summerhill or some other special school. Dr. Feller advised the Frumkins against sending her to such a school, because "she shouldn't have that stigma in later life." She recommended a small coeducational private school in Flushing, a short bus ride from the Frumkins' house in Beechhurst. Sylvia could get up in the morning at seven-forty-five and easily get to school by nine. School let out at two-thirty in the afternoon, so she could avoid traveling home in the evening rush hour. Harriet Frumkin telephoned the school, explained Sylvia's situation to the director, and asked if the school would consider admitting her. The director asked her to send him Sylvia's transcript from Music and Art. After receiving it, he accepted her without a test or an interview. Sylvia Frumkin was discharged from Creedmoor on October 22, 1964. A few days later, she started the eleventh grade at the new school, a month behind her classmates. Sylvia did well there academically. She was good in history, French, and English. She was asked to drop chemistry, however, because she was clumsy. Her chemistry teacher told her, only half jokingly, that he was afraid she would blow up the chemistry lab. Sylvia liked the school's small classes — there were only twelve or thirteen students in each section of history and English — but she found her new classmates less bright than her classmates at Music and Art had been, and in her opinion many of them were rich snobs.

In the 1950s and 1960s, it was the custom for young middle-class girls in Queens to be given lavish sixteenth-birthday celebrations. Joyce Frumkin had had her Sweet Sixteen party at an expensive restaurant. On May 5, 1965, because Sylvia had spent her sixteenth birthday at St. Vincent's Hospital, the Frumkins gave her a Sweet Seventeen party. Harriet Frumkin's favorite color, like Sylvia's, is pink. She had been married in a pink dress, a pink hat, and pink shoes. For Sylvia's party, the Frumkins chose a restaurant that had a room painted pink. The china, the glasses, the tablecloths and napkins, the cake, Sylvia's dress and corsage, and the corsages for the seventeen girls who had been invited to the party were pink. Most of the guests, who had received pink invitations, were the girls in her new eleventh-grade class. A few were former classmates from Music and Art. Camilla Costello did not receive an invitation to the party. Sylvia had telephoned Camilla from Creedmoor a number of times during her stay there. Mrs. Costello had threatened to sue the hospital if Sylvia made any further attempts to get in touch with her daughter. The Frumkins were informed of Mrs. Costello's threats, and had to tell Sylvia not to call Camilla again. Sylvia was never to make a friend she cared about as much as she had cared for Camilla.

Each Saturday morning during Sylvia's first year at the school in Flushing, Mr. Frumkin drove her to Bayside, where Ida Feller lived, for a session of psychotherapy. Miss Frumkin recalls Dr. Feller as a pleasant woman — but one to whom she couldn't relate. Just as Camilla Costello was the only friend she ever had who mattered to her, Francine Baden was the only therapist with whom she would ever try to work out her problems. "With Francine, something just clicked," she said recently. For the next seventeen years, she would talk longingly, though often ambivalently, about Miss Baden. "She helped me in the short run with everything from the way I looked to the way I thought about myself," she would say. "But perhaps she hurt me in the long run, by making me rebel against my parents. Maybe she opened Pandora's box." Dr. Feller was the first of many therapists Sylvia saw after Miss Baden with whom nothing clicked. When Sylvia discussed her behavior with Dr. Feller — for example, when she told her that she had pushed her mother or had twisted her mother's arm — Dr. Feller scolded her for being violent. She didn't explore with Sylvia the reasons for her violent behavior.

There were times in 1965 when the Frumkins thought that

Sylvia's troubles were over — that what she had had in 1964 was just "a nervous episode," as Dr. Feller had put it. Sylvia sang with a community chorus one evening a week, she behaved politely at her Sweet Seventeen party, she got good grades at school. Still, there were times when something brought them up short. One day after school, Sylvia called home. Her mother answered the telephone. Her father was still at work. Sylvia said she was in a telephone booth and didn't remember how to get home. Mrs. Frumkin asked Sylvia to describe the location of the phone booth, and told her to stay where she was. She took a bus to Flushing and found Sylvia huddled up in a booth and looking so frightened that Mrs. Frumkin thought she must have seen demons. At first, she could say only, "Mommy, I'm scared." Mrs. Frumkin took her home on the bus. And Joyce Frumkin recalls, "Even in a good year, there were troubles with Sylvia. There was the pinching and the shoving."

⁊ ⁊ ⁊

In June of 1965, Benjamin Wilder came to New York on a business trip. He was then chairman of the biology department at a college in Chicago, where he taught courses and also supervised a research laboratory. He came to Beechhurst and was chagrined to see his mother reigning over the household from the master bedroom the Frumkins had given her, and to see Sylvia tyrannizing over the household with her temper tantrums. Wilder considered Harriet and Irving Frumkin weak people who simply let Sylvia get away with unacceptable behavior. Some years earlier, on learning that when Sylvia threatened to throw up in the car she was given a bag instead of a sound spanking, he had concluded that she was a spoiled brat. He also faulted both Frumkins as parents in other ways — Irving for idolizing Joyce at Sylvia's expense, and his sister for devoting too much time to art lessons and too little time to Sylvia. Benjamin Wilder and his wife, Judith, had two children — a daughter, Dorothy, who was Joyce's age and was studying in California, and a son, Seth, who was Sylvia's age. Benjamin Wilder took pride in his happy marriage and his well-brought-up children, neither of whom had ever smashed up a car or been in a psychiatric hospital. He flew home and asked Judith if she was willing to have Sylvia spend July and August with them at their home, in Chicago. When she said that she was, he invited Sylvia to come to Chicago to work in his laboratory. He flew to New York to get her several weeks later. Sylvia was excited about going to Chicago; she had never been on an airplane. As he flew with his niece to Chicago, Benjamin Wilder was convinced that she was merely the product of a bad environment and would therefore be helped merely by being put in a good environment. "I'll send you home a well girl," he told his sister at the airport.

The Wilders gave Sylvia a few days to adjust to her new surroundings. Then Benjamin Wilder told Sylvia that the time had come for her to start work. The night before she was to go to the laboratory for the first time, she was in a near-frenzy. She clearly did not want to go to work. Her uncle believed that she was fearful of facing a new situation, and tried to allay her anxiety while saying firmly that she was going to go to the lab. Sylvia was supposed to be dressed and ready to leave for the lab at seven o'clock the next morning. She procrastinated. Her uncle told her to hurry. When she finally got dressed and came downstairs, she said she had to take her Thorazine tablets with her. She went back upstairs, came down again, and spilled the tablets all over the living-room floor. "If you think you're going to get out of going to the lab this way, you're mistaken," he told his niece. "Get down on your hands and knees, pick up as many tablets as you need, and get in the car." Benjamin Wilder had told his chief lab technician that Sylvia had had some problems; the other lab employees knew only that she was the boss's niece. On her third day in the lab, Sylvia dropped an expensive beaker. Her uncle believed that she had dropped it on purpose. He showed her how to sweep up the glass fragments without getting hurt, and she did. From then on, she worked well at the lab. She got along with her coworkers and earned the salary she was paid.

Sylvia did not do nearly as well outside the lab. Her uncle drove her to the lab each morning, but several evenings a week he stayed late to teach a summer-school course. Sylvia's workday ended at four o'clock, and she was supposed to take a bus back to the Wilders' home directly after work. Instead, she started wandering around Chicago, using her lab earnings to buy a great deal of rouge and lipstick, and often came home late. Weekends, when the Wilders had made plans for outings with their friends and Seth's friends, in which Sylvia was included, she tended to wander off by herself. Judith Wilder believed that Sylvia realized she couldn't be like normal teen-agers and therefore tried to avoid them. At home with just her aunt, uncle, and cousin, Sylvia was often defiant. When it was time to eat dinner, she said she wanted to stay in her room; she threw temper tantrums when her uncle insisted that she come to the table. The Wilders owned a Doberman pinscher named Bandit. The dog didn't usually take to strangers, but he liked Sylvia. Wilder warned Sylvia never to take the dog out alone, though, because he was strong, and hard to control on a leash. One day while her uncle was out, Sylvia took Bandit out alone. The dog lunged and got away from her, leash and all. When she returned home without the dog, her uncle was there. She told him what had happened. He shouted at her for having disobeyed him.

"You know, when people shout at me I can be violent!" Sylvia shouted back.

"What do you mean?" her uncle asked.

"I've been in mental hospitals, so I can be violent and I can't be held responsible for what I might do to you."

Wilder told Sylvia that if he ever heard her say anything

like that again he would beat her to a pulp. He insisted that she accompany him to search for Bandit. It took them an hour to find the dog. When they did, Wilder told Sylvia to take the leash and not let go of it. She refused — Wilder had the feeling that she didn't want to try again and fail again — so he told the dog to heel, and they walked home. Sylvia didn't take the dog out a second time. Wilder, who acknowledges that he is an impatient man with a quick temper, did not slap Sylvia on that occasion, but he did slap her a few days later, for using obscene language, which he would not permit his own children to use. Sylvia seemed stunned at being the slapped rather than the slapper. She was supposed to stay with the Wilders for nine weeks. After five weeks, Wilder bought her a plane ticket to New York, called the Frumkins, and told them he was sending Sylvia home.

When Benjamin Wilder reminisced recently about Sylvia's summer in Chicago, he said he could have tolerated Sylvia's presence in his home for a few more weeks if he had had to, but that she was taking such a toll on him that he had asked himself whether it was his mission in life to fight with her every day to make her behave acceptably. His answer to that question was no. He felt that if she had stayed with him much longer he would have lost his mind. In 1981, Wilder, who doesn't believe that genetics or chemical imbalances have anything to do with his niece's illness, regretted only one thing: having to send Sylvia back to her parents. "I'd much rather have sent Sylvia to the Mojave Desert than to the environment that produced her," he said. "She knew just how to manipulate her parents. At home, she could escape responsibility, and if she wanted to escape even further into madness she could go to a mental institution and be crazy there to her heart's content, because people would have to put up with her."

When Wilder called his sister to tell her he was sending Sylvia home early, Mrs. Frumkin didn't seem displeased. Her brother had an explanation for that, too. "Harriet was crippled by our overbearing mother," he says. "It makes her feel less of a cripple to be surrounded by other cripples. That's why she married Irving Frumkin. They've always seemed to me to be two cripples who were more comfortable being miserable together than being miserable apart. Their marriage requires Sylvia's illness to divert them from their own miseries. Taking in my mother and, after her death, taking in my mother's awful sister Lottie were further masochistic diversions. Harriet and Irving have a terrific investment in Sylvia's illness. It gives their lives a purpose. I don't think they would survive if Sylvia ever got well." The statements made by Wilder have also been made by any number of psychiatrists, psychologists, social workers, and attendants who have known Sylvia and her parents over the past seventeen years.

⸙ ⸙ ⸙

Sylvia Frumkin did not return home from Chicago a well girl. When she flew home, she was too agitated for the Frumkins to handle. Shock treatments had worked a miracle on her at Creedmoor, so her parents took her to a doctor who gave ECT to patients in his office, in Kew Gardens, Queens. Sylvia calmed down after several shock treatments and was able to start the twelfth grade with her classmates in September.

After completing the shock treatments, Sylvia Frumkin said that she felt fine and didn't want to see a psychiatrist for therapy. The Frumkins told her that if she wouldn't see a therapist she would have to return to Creedmoor. Sylvia said she didn't want to go back to Dr. Feller. A friend had told the Frumkins about a psychiatrist in the Bronx, Dr. Max Brunner. They made an appointment for Sylvia to meet him. She agreed to go to see him on Saturdays.

Sylvia Frumkin found Dr. Brunner as unhelpful as Dr. Feller had been. When she told him how much her classmates disliked her, he didn't seem properly sympathetic.

"They are not part of your future," he said sternly. She frequently broke appointments with him without telling her parents, who were not pleased to pay for missed sessions. Dr. Brunner raised Sylvia's daily medication from 300 milligrams of Thorazine to 300 milligrams of Thorazine and 30 milligrams of Stelazine, roughly equivalent to 900 milligrams of Thorazine — a maintenance dose that is adequate for many patients.

Because Sylvia Frumkin felt that she had little in common with her classmates — many of them the sons and daughters of wealthy doctors and businessmen, whose wealth she resented and envied — she joined the YM-YWHA in Flushing. There she met a group of less affluent teen-agers, with whom she felt more at ease. Joyce had taught her how to play the guitar. Sylvia was popular when she played her guitar at the Y in the fall of 1965. Each winter, the Flushing Y had a talent contest for teen-agers. In January of 1966, Sylvia was nominated and became one of ten finalists. On the afternoon of the contest, she was all set to sing and accompany herself on the guitar at the Y that evening. She had a date, a new pink dress, and a corsage her date had sent her. A few hours before the contest was to begin, she ran away. She came home the following day. She remembered few details about the episode, but she did later acknowledge that she had run away because the pressure of competition was too great for her and she was afraid that she would lose the contest. Sylvia had returned home distraught. The Frumkins called the doctor in Kew Gardens who had given her shock treatments in his office the previous August. He admitted her to a hospital in Kew Gardens, where he gave her a series of shock treatments. She was able to return to school, although the shock treatments were not as effective as they had been in the past. Sylvia became progressively more agitated in the spring.

Most of Sylvia's classmates were planning to go to college. In the fall of her senior year, Sylvia was considering going to an out-of-town college, as her sister had done. Mr. Frumkin had driven Joyce around to look at the colleges to which she had applied. In the fall of 1965, he drove Sylvia to see Bard College, in Annandale-on-Hudson — a school with a good name in the fine arts. Sylvia had an interview at Bard, whose reputation for being unstructured appealed to her, but she never filled out the lengthy application form for the college. "I didn't have the strength," she said recently. She applied to Hunter College, then one of New York City's five tuition-free four-year colleges, which admitted graduates of the city's high schools who had high averages. Sylvia wasn't just accepted at Hunter; she was accepted into the college honors program for outstanding students.

Toward the end of twelfth grade, her condition worsened. She was excused from final exams, but she graduated with her class, on June 15, 1966. A snapshot taken by her father on graduation day shows a slightly heavy young woman in a cap and gown, wearing a tense expression. While Sylvia was at Creedmoor in 1964, she had weighed between 130 and 133 pounds. In June of 1966, she weighed 146 pounds. One of the many unpleasant side effects of neuroleptics is a gain in weight — a major reason that so many patients stop taking the medication prescribed for them.

During the spring of her senior year, when Sylvia's classmates spoke of going to Penn State or to the University of Miami, Sylvia often said she was going to Hillside instead of saying she was going to Hunter. She often spoke to her parents of her wish to go to Hillside. Her friend Arlene Epstein, who had spent six weeks there in 1962, had gone right back to high school from Hillside and was now doing well as a freshman in college. Whenever Sylvia said she wished to go to Hillside, her parents told her to concentrate on graduating from high school.

After her graduation, Sylvia stayed in her room a lot; she slept a great deal, and she played her records for hours. One day, she went by bus to Hillside Hospital and spoke to a resident there. She discussed her psychiatric history with him, and said she wanted to go to Hillside for six weeks "to psych up" for Hunter. He encouraged her to apply for admission. She came home and told her parents about the interview. She said that she was exhausted and that Hillside looked like the perfect place for her to rest up before college. The Frumkins were opposed to Sylvia's going to Hillside. They called Dr. Brunner, who was also opposed to her going to a hospital, but neither he nor the Frumkins could convince Sylvia that she was better off receiving treatment as an outpatient. She kept pleading with her parents until they finally consented to her admission. Hillside was a hospital that accepted only voluntary patients, and was noted for its emphasis on research and training. It had almost two hundred in-patients, about half of them housed in pleasant, unlocked cottages. The average length of stay at Hillside in 1966 was six months, but some patients were kept for more than a year if the hospital was satisfied with their progress. At Hillside, the ratio of psychiatric residents to patients was high enough that patients could see their doctors frequently, and there were therapeutic programs scheduled from one end of the day to the other. The hospital was selective: Chronic patients were screened out.

Sylvia Frumkin was admitted to Hillside on June 22, 1966, exactly a week after her graduation from high school. She was experiencing auditory hallucinations (voices directed her to perform acts like lighting a cigarette); she was in what the admitting doctor termed "a disorganized state." She was put in a semiprivate room and was immediately taken off her medication — Dr. Brunner's daily dosage of 300 milligrams of Thorazine and 30 milligrams of Stelazine. This was the customary procedure at Hillside. The doctors wanted whatever medication was in a patient's bloodstream to wash out, so that they could see the patient's psychosis for themselves, diagnose it accurately, and then treat it appropriately. Many psychiatrists approve of this practice, especially if length and cost of hospitalization are not major concerns and if hospitals are well staffed with attendants and nurses who are willing to cope with unmedicated patients — conditions that rarely exist nowadays.

Sylvia Frumkin was kept off medication at Hillside for three weeks. She became progressively more agitated and delusional. After three weeks, she was put back on medication: Her daily dose was soon 4000 milligrams of Thorazine and 15 milligrams of Stelazine (the equivalent of 4300 milligrams of Thorazine). Because Hillside emphasized research, such high doses of neuroleptics were not unheard of there in 1966. Though most patients responded to 1800 milligrams of Thorazine a day, those who didn't were given as much as 5000 milligrams; most responded to these doses, which were far above the ones recommended by the drug manufacturers in the *Physicians' Desk Reference.* One nurse who took care of Sylvia Frumkin at Hillside in 1966 remembers that the high dose of medication had no apparent effect on her. A nurse couldn't even enter Miss Frumkin's room alone. She believed she was a cat, and clawed at anyone who came near her; nurses had to be sent to her room in pairs. Her condition continued to deteriorate; she became more and more hyperactive, confused, and delusional.

In September, Miss Frumkin was taken off Thorazine and Stelazine and was put on Librium, an anti-anxiety drug. She became more aggressive and argumentative, and exhibited bizarre behavior, such as undressing in the middle of the cottage — "to be the way God made me," as she put it. The specialist in psychopharmacology who recently reviewed her medical record was not favorably impressed by the treatment she received at Hillside in 1966. "Taking her off medication was a good idea, but I think she should have been put back on medication before her symptoms became so florid," he said. "You can diagnose patients accurately and treat them intelligently without seeing them at their worst. It's damaging to patients to let them become too sick, because that grave sickness will become part of their self-image, and that can have a negative effect on their future. Librium is not an antipsychotic. One of the side effects of Librium and Valium in susceptible individuals is paradoxical rage — the drugs that are supposed to calm people release their anger."

Sylvia Frumkin was far too ill to enjoy Hillside as she had expected to. She quarreled with her roommate. She was unable to go on the camping trips and trips to amusement parks that had been planned. She regarded activities like flower arranging as "intellectually unstimulating," and couldn't concentrate on any form of occupational or recreational therapy. One day in late September, she walked out of her cottage. She went to Greenwich Village, a neighborhood she had enjoyed during her year and a half at Music and Art. She telephoned Joyce in the middle of the night and said she was in a storefront crash pad near Bleecker Street. Joyce met her there and took her to a coffee shop that stayed open all night. Sylvia was surprisingly calm. She told Joyce about two men she had slept with in the crash pad. They talked until dawn. After breakfast, Sylvia said she was willing to return to Hillside. Joyce drove her back. Upon her return, Sylvia requested ECT. Hillside started to give her a series of shock treatments in mid-October. For a few days after her first three shock treatments, her behavior improved; then she became agitated, confused, extremely disorganized, violently argumentative, and aggressive. She fought with the staff, she undressed in the cottage, and she expressed delusions of persecution.

Like St. Vincent's, Hillside preferred "good" patients. Sylvia Frumkin was informed that she could no longer stay at Hillside and that she would be transferred to Creedmoor. She refused to go there voluntarily. Her plan had been to go from Hillside to Hunter in the fall, and not from Hillside to Creedmoor. Two psychiatrists at Hillside examined Miss Frumkin and certified that she was dangerous to herself and others and therefore required further, involuntary hospitalization. She was sent from Hillside to Creedmoor on October 27, 1966, on what was known as a two-physicians' certificate, or a two P.C., which was valid for sixty days. Her diagnosis was schizophrenia, chronic undifferentiated. (*Chronic undifferentiated* is a term applied loosely to schizophrenics who have been ill for a long time, because as the illness progresses and the personality deteriorates the symptoms become less clear-cut.) She screamed in the ambulance during the short ride from Hillside to Creedmoor. She probably would have screamed louder if she had had any idea that by the time she next got out of Creedmoor her private-school classmates would be midway through their junior year in college.

Fifteen

The doctor in Building 40 who screened Miss Frumkin for admission on October 27, 1966, was not required to admit her — he could, on the basis of his own assessment of her condition, have recommended that she return home and be treated as an out-patient — but in 1966 Creedmoor hardly ever turned a patient away. The doctor who interviewed Miss Frumkin and admitted her to Ward 10-A noted "profuse, rambling, and pointlessly digressive" expressions and "fragmented associations." Miss Frumkin acknowledged having recently experienced auditory hallucinations (a voice had told her to strip her clothes off at Hillside), but she denied hearing any voices on October 27. She was fully oriented, and her memory was intact. The doctor found her affect dominated by an "intense, all-pervasive rage. She had to be forcibly taken to the ward." The doctor's tentative diagnosis was schizophrenia, undifferentiated type.

According to the notes that the attendants wrote about Miss Frumkin on October 27 and October 28, she was hostile, belligerent to employees and other patients, and sarcastic. When she was asked to give a urine specimen, she threw some bedpans on the floor. When she was asked to get dressed, she said, "I will not until I get good and ready," and paraded up and down the hallway undressed, demanding to see a doctor and a social worker. She was sent to 11-A, the ward for aggressive patients, on October 28 — much sooner than she had been after her 1964 admission. On October 31, shortly after her return from 11-A, an attendant wrote a progress note on her that was similar in both its content and its tone to most of the notes that were written about her between 1966 and 1981: "Pt. remains uncooperative and is very pesty. Inconsiderate of others, expects partial treatment and expects employees to cater to her impulsive whims. Quite annoying; does not appear to be well liked by other patients on ward because of her attitude of superiority."

Although Mr. Frumkin requested on October 30 that Sylvia be given electroshock treatment, she was instead given moderate doses of Mellaril or of Thorazine and Stelazine during all of November and December. The doses never exceeded the equivalent of 800 milligrams of Thorazine. In the mid-sixties, Creedmoor was still giving doses that were too low to allay Miss Frumkin's agitation and excitement. Her parents were told not to visit her. Other relatives, who upset her less — among them Joyce Frumkin and Phyllis Frumkin — were permitted to visit and did. In December, Sylvia applied for admission to Creedmoor's insulin unit.

In the late 1920s, a Viennese psychiatrist named Manfred Sakel had noticed that an overdose of insulin given to a drug addict appeared to alleviate the addict's withdrawal symptoms. Sakel started treating schizophrenics with overdoses of insulin — deliberately putting them into comas, which insulin overdoses cause, and then reviving them. He claimed to have good results. Insulin-coma therapy, or ICT, was introduced at Creedmoor in 1937. Patients were given large doses of insulin to reduce their blood-sugar level and induce coma. After an hour or so, the patients were revived with large amounts of glucose. In 1951, Dr. Sheldon Jolis, a Belgian immigrant who had just finished his residency at Creedmoor, took charge of the hospital's insulin unit. By December of 1966, when Miss Frumkin was admitted to the insulin unit, most psychiatrists had come to believe that the antipsychotic drugs made ICT obsolete.

Dr. Jolis did not share that opinion, although he was not really interested in insulin per se. His objective, as he explained in his writings for professional journals, was to use the Creedmoor insulin unit as a base on which to build an ideal "therapeutic community" — one that combined the best of physical treatments for schizophrenia with the best of psychotherapy. The rough outline of his theory is held by a number of other psychiatrists. These psychiatrists believe that neither their biologically oriented colleagues of the "nature school" nor the psychoanalysts and psychotherapists of the "nurture school" have developed an adequate approach to mental illness. They are convinced that the optimum treatment — insofar as one can be devised on the basis of the limited knowledge of mental illness — is to attempt to correct both nature and nurture. The first step is to diagnose the illness correctly and to bring the psychosis under control with drug therapy. Then an attempt is made to keep the patient on an adequate maintenance dose while using individual psychotherapy to try to give the patient self-understanding and skills to cope with everyday life. Some schizophrenics — those who are too withdrawn or too willful or who feel too threatened — cannot be reached by psychotherapy. These psychiatrists feel that psychotherapy is particularly important for schizophrenics who are receptive to it, because the disease has subterranean symptoms as destructive as the hallucinations and delusions that are among its overt ones. The drugs can bring the positive symptoms of schizophrenia under control, but they cannot touch the negative ones, such as the inability to socialize or to experience pleasure. Only psychotherapy can ameliorate these symptoms. In severe cases like Miss Frumkin's, individual psychotherapy would have to be given several times a week, and the process would be a long and tedious one, because a medication-resistant schizophrenic is likely to be just as resistant to psychotherapy.

Miss Frumkin had never received this optimum treatment of a simultaneous combination of proper medication and effective psychotherapy. Dr. Jolis said that he was going to give it to her. He did not promise to cure schizophrenia, but he offered the next best thing — "social recovery" of the patient. He said that his mode of treatment was expressly designed to take "chronic cases" and turn them into functioning human beings who could live in the community. Dr. Jolis did not rely only on insulin-coma therapy for the physical-treatment side of his "therapeutic community." He varied the physical remedies in accordance with what he saw to be the needs of the patient. To some he gave ICT alone; to others a combination of electroshock and drugs, and no ICT; and to still others ICT, ECT, and drugs. For the nonphysical side, he did not give individual psychotherapy. He said that it made schizophrenics dependent on their therapist without solving their problems. Instead, he used a form of group therapy called multifamily therapy, or MFT. This was particularly efficacious in schizophrenia, Dr. Jolis wrote, explaining, "The locus of illness is the family rather than the individual . . . The patient's illness not only affects significant others in his environment but is often perpetuated by them . . . If lasting improvement in the patient's condition is to be achieved, his home environment has to be changed. His family have to become more accepting of him and communications between the patient and all members of his family must be improved or restored." The therapy groups consisted of four or five schizophrenics and their families, and were arranged so that each group met once a week for an hour and a quarter. Dr. Jolis led most of the therapy sessions himself. He also employed a psychiatric social worker in the insulin unit, who held occasional private therapy sessions with an individual schizophrenic and his or her family to reinforce what had been said in the group meetings.

Dr. Jolis's unique approach to schizophrenia permitted him

to transform the insulin unit at Creedmoor into an elite enclave. By using ICT at a time when it was rapidly losing ground to drugs, he obtained grants from the Manfred Sakel Foundation, in Manhattan, which sought to perpetuate the work of the originator of insulin therapy; and his multifamily therapy enabled him to obtain further funds, in generous amounts, from government sources. In 1981, Creedmoor employees who had been at the hospital in December of 1966, when Miss Frumkin entered the insulin unit, recalled that it had been the most agreeable-looking place in the hospital. It had the nicest furniture, the most abundant supplies for recreational and occupational therapy, the most space per patient, and the most staff per patient. The fact that the insulin unit, on the second floor, was far better funded than any of the other floors in Building 40, not to mention the back-ward buildings, and was thus luxurious by comparison, made many patients want to be in it or caused their families to urge their admission. Dr. Jolis selected his patients carefully, however. They had to be between the ages of seventeen and thirty-five, show what he considered an adequate level of intelligence, and have either a spouse or parents who were willing to make regular financial contributions to the insulin unit, take part in the weekly sessions of MFT, and consent to the filming of some sessions. The films were used to raise additional funds. Harriet and Irving Frumkin made a weekly contribution and also helped, as the other families did, to raise more money by holding auctions and fairs. Dr. Jolis is also remembered for selecting his staff carefully: All his nurses were pretty. There were television sets and phonographs for the patients, special movies and outings, and special visiting hours. Relatives of patients in the insulin unit could visit frequently; families of patients in the rest of the hospital were allowed to visit only on Wednesday and Sunday afternoons.

Late in December, Miss Frumkin was moved from Ward 10-A to Ward 2-A, the insulin ward. In January of 1967, she was given small doses of insulin, to see if she could tolerate it, and 450 milligrams of Thorazine and 20 milligrams of Stelazine (the equivalent of 850 milligrams of Thorazine), to control her behavior. Like many patients, she found the insulin doses unpleasant. On January 11, 1967, according to a note on her chart, she had "to be forced to insulin area daily." On the eleventh, thirteenth, and sixteenth of January, she was therefore given ECT treatments "to control her impulsive and aggressive behavior." She responded favorably to these: She stopped attacking the attendants and fighting with the other patients in the unit, and she became more receptive to insulin. From January until April, she was given doses of insulin three times a week to determine the optimum dose. Then, between April and December of 1967, she was given thirty-five insulin comas. On those thirty-five mornings, she was put to bed and injected with insulin until she went into a hypoglycemic coma. Nurses and attendants remained at her bedside to check her vital signs. Dr. Jolis had developed a monitoring system that resembled traffic lights and could be controlled manually. If the patient was in a safe coma, the nurses and attendants kept a green light on. If the patient went into a medium-deep coma, they turned on a yellow light. If the patient's vital signs indicated that he or she had gone into a dangerously deep coma, a red light was turned on, and a doctor terminated the coma. Patients in yellow and green comas were revived with glucagon after an hour of unconsciousness. They often needed additional doses of glucagon when they felt weak later on.

Dr. Jolis made two basic assumptions in his approach to schizophrenia. The first was that, despite what he conceded to be "the absence of precise knowledge of the causes of mental illness," he knew how to bring the psychosis under control by selectively or collectively applying insulin shock, electroshock, and drugs. Harriet and Irving Frumkin remember that their daughter's condition improved in 1967, but the monthly notes kept by the unit's doctors and attendants indicate that her progress was irregular and uncertain:

April: friendly and cooperative, but is still very agitated . . . She leaves her personal belongings all over the ward and is quite disorganized in her thinking and actions.

May: Pt. feels no one likes her & people are only friendly toward her when it meets their needs. Feels as though she is the scapegoat of the ward. Pt. is fidgety, pulls at her hair & picks at her lip.

June: Pt.'s appearance remains slovenly, cannot sit still for any period of time, speaks rapidly & jumps from one topic to another. For a large part of the day, Sylvia sits in front of the TV.

Sept: Her behavior is erratic, and she is often flamboyant, boisterous, and disruptive.

Nov: She has recently participated in the ward variety show with great success. . . . Patient continues to improve.

Dr. Jolis's second basic assumption was that although the family of a treatment-resistant schizophrenic might be as resistant to therapy as the schizophrenic, the technique of multifamily therapy would break down the family's resistance and change the family environment so that "recurrence can be prevented." He wrote of his second assumption in an article in 1961, "It is almost certain that these sessions will to a degree modify the home environment to which the patient eventually will return." Of the numerous sessions of MFT that the Frumkins attended, one session stands out in their memory. Dr. Jolis was at the front of a room filled with patients and their relatives. Miss Frumkin was sitting next to her mother. Her nose was running. She reached into her mother's pocket, found a Kleenex there, and used it to blow her nose. Dr. Jolis had observed this scene. He stopped talking in midsentence and called the incident to the attention of the others present. "I want you to note the interaction between Sylvia and her mother," he told the gathering. "Sylvia needed a Kleenex or a handkerchief. Instead of getting up and going to get one from her room, she got one out of her mother's pocket. There you have a perfect example of a symbiotic relationship."

Another hospital staff member in the room, who wasn't sure that this kind of holding people up as public examples had quite the effect Dr. Jolis thought it did, noticed that Mrs. Frumkin looked pleased to have been singled out for special attention, and did not seem vulnerable to the dart that Dr. Jolis had tossed her way. "What's this nonsense about symbiotic relationships?" Mrs. Frumkin said boldly. "All Sylvia wanted was a Kleenex because her nose was running."

Dr. Jolis believed in being direct with his patients. He once told a former patient in the insulin unit — a suicidal young man who had threatened to jump out a window — "It's up to you, but if you decide you don't want to live, for God's sake don't jump out the window. You might fail and end up a cripple, and then you'd be worse. Just take pills and do a good job." The following year, the patient took an overdose of barbiturates and died.

The therapy sessions that the Frumkins and Sylvia had with the psychiatric social worker in the insulin unit, Janet Poster, did not proceed as cordially as the MFT sessions with Dr. Jolis. Mrs. Poster held many therapy sessions with Sylvia and her parents in 1967 and early 1968. She often had to see Sylvia with either her father or her mother, because Mr. and Mrs. Frumkin fought with each other so much that Mrs. Poster could seldom accomplish anything when both of them were in the room. Mrs. Frumkin, Mrs. Poster, and Sylvia remember one session in which the three of them were in Mrs. Poster's office. When Sylvia was in junior high school, she had read a collection of short stories dealing with personal fantasies. One story was about a distant planet called Verna. Life was simpler and more serene on Verna than on earth. There was less pressure and drudgery, so people on Verna had more time to do the things they wanted. A few people from earth could arrange to be transported to Verna. Sylvia wanted to be one of them. Sometimes she imagined she was already there. During that particular session, she was fantasizing about being on Verna.

Mrs. Poster was upset. She wanted to get Sylvia to face reality, not to evade it. "Cut out the nonsense about Verna — you're right here with me in this office," she said. "This is the real world. Come back from the make-believe."

Sylvia looked at her and said, "Mrs. Poster, you live in the real world, and my parents live in the real world. I'd prefer to live in an imaginary place like Verna. In my world, I can be anyone I want to be. But what does your world have to offer me, Mrs. Poster? In your world, I'm nothing."

Mrs. Poster did not have any theories about the causes of schizophrenia. When she was once asked about schizophrenogenic mothers, genetic predispositions, and biochemical imbalances, she said, "I really don't know." What she firmly believed was that when a person like Sylvia Frumkin came down with the illness, "the family had some real influence in making it better or worse." Like so many other people who had treated or known Miss Frumkin, and like so many who were to treat her or know her later, Mrs. Poster had a lot of sympathy for her, because of her parents. She found the Frumkins even more difficult than the parents of most other schizophrenic patients she saw regularly. Almost all the parents were difficult, however, as Mrs. Poster would have expected them to be. Mrs. Poster knew a lot about the emotional toll of working with schizophrenics for a few hours a day. She could imagine the consequences of living with them.

Far from feeling like one of a fortunate hundred out of thousands of patients in Creedmoor because she was in the insulin unit, Sylvia Frumkin remembers her many months there as among the worst in her life. Like most other patients in the unit, she gained a great deal of weight as a result of the glucose. She had come to Creedmoor in October of 1966 weighing 146 pounds. By August of 1967, she weighed 178 pounds. She also dreaded the comas; they were frightening and gave her a desperate sense of helplessness. In December of 1967, Miss Frumkin developed a serious upper-respiratory infection. Her insulin treatments were stopped while her infection was treated with antibiotics. She was considered by a doctor to be "in good contact with reality." On December 13, she wrote a letter to Dr. Jolis in which she pleaded to be taken off insulin. "I am nothing but a malingering fraud," she wrote. "I am not sick enough to be here. I will go to Dr. Brunner and get well on the outside. I am sure of it."

In 1967, the minimum number of insulin comas that Dr. Jolis wanted his patients to have was forty. (In earlier years, he had written articles advocating ninety comas if forty or seventy were ineffective.) In January, in part because Miss Frumkin had had only thirty-five comas and in part because while she was off insulin she had started to get auditory and visual hallucinations, she was put back on ICT. On February 13, the day she had her fortieth coma, she again wrote to the insulin-unit staff begging to be let off insulin now that she had completed fifteen yellow and twenty-five green comas. She said she felt that insulin had done all it could for her. She said she wanted to take typing and stenography or home economics at Creedmoor; get a job, an apartment, and her discharge; start taking college courses in the fall of 1968 and return to college full time in July of 1969. She was allowed to stop taking insulin on February 27, because her thinking was "clearer" and her doctor approved of her plans, but she remained in the insulin unit. She continued to participate in family-therapy sessions and to go on insulin-unit trips, and she started to attend homemaking classes. Her medication varied from month to month. In March of 1968, she received Thorazine and Stelazine; in April, Taractan; and in May, Haldol. All her doses of these drugs were the equivalent of about three hundred milligrams of Thorazine.

The specialist in psychopharmacology who recently reviewed Miss Frumkin's record said of her stay at Creedmoor in 1967 and 1968, "First, she was given insulin-coma therapy, which by then was considered outmoded and dangerous. No really well-controlled studies comparing it to other forms of treatment were done. I'm convinced that insulin often messed up patients' metabolisms for the rest of their lives. Once Miss Frumkin was taken off insulin, she was given sub-therapeutic doses of a variety of drugs. At that time, some doctors dispensed drugs the way they might flick TV channels when all the programs were boring."

On Saturday, April 13, 1968, while Miss Frumkin was home for the weekend, she became agitated and disturbed. She left the house. Her father went out in his car to look for her. He found her several hours later, walking around aimlessly a few blocks away, and coaxed her into the car. As he was driving her home, she jumped from the moving vehicle, fell, and suffered minor injuries. He drove her back to the hospital, where her wounds were cleaned and dressed. She had a one-inch cut under her chin, which required three stitches, and an abrasion on her left knee. She was acutely psychotic when she returned to the insulin unit. She broke a phonograph record in the dayhall that evening, because, she said, it was "an evil record" and she couldn't stand the sound of it. The next day, she talked about hearing voices, "such as Paul McCartney of the Beatles"; about having got into a YMCA "the other night"; and about wanting to see Creedmoor's Protestant minister to change her religion. On April 19, she fought with several other patients; on April 20, she kept taking her clothes off; on April 21, she was sent to Ward 11-A for two days. In late April, she was so nasty to the other patients in the insulin unit that they threatened to harm her if she didn't stop annoying them. On May 4, she was sent to 11-A again. On May 6, she returned to 2-A "as nasty as ever." On May 10, she chased another female patient in 2-A, saying that the patient was a boy and that she was in love with him. Between May 22 and June 19, Miss Frumkin received twelve ECT treatments, "because of extreme agitation and psychotic thinking." After the course of ECT, she was found to be "more coherent and under greater control." Her thinking was "somewhat clearer."

⁄ ⁄ ⁄

At four o'clock on the afternoon of Thursday, June 27, Miss Frumkin went with the other members of the insulin unit to a barbecue in the recreation room of Building 40. She left the barbecue without anyone's noticing her departure. That evening, Mrs. Frumkin telephoned the insulin unit to say she had received a call from a Catholic priest at a church in Flushing, who had told her that Sylvia was with him in his rectory. After notifying the hospital, Mrs. Frumkin and a friend went to the church, where they waited for three Creedmoor employees who had been sent there to take Sylvia back to the hospital. She returned to the hospital reluctantly. Upon her return, she said she was tired of Creedmoor; otherwise, she talked in riddles and was incoherent, irrelevant, and nervous. On June 29, she was very disturbed, and said she was turning into a cat. Whenever anyone opened a door, she tried to escape. On June 30, she was sent to Ward 11-A.

During the first two weeks of July, Sylvia Frumkin became increasingly confused. She provoked fights, and she slept on the floor of the insulin ward, to which she had been returned. On July 16, a doctor in the insulin unit wrote that "she has become increasingly more unmanageable on this ward and arrangements have been made for her transfer to Building R." From the time it opened, in 1936, Building R had housed Creedmoor's "most disturbed" women patients. Along with Building S, the building for Creedmoor's "most disturbed" men patients, it was one of the most terrifying places in the hospital. There were constant assaults in Building R; it was noisy, overcrowded, and foul-smelling. On July 18, to make room for a yet more disturbed patient, Miss Frumkin was transferred from Building R to Building O — a "continued treatment" building that dated from the 1920s. She had been given 200 milligrams of Thorazine during her two days in Building R. During her four weeks in Building O, which was then primarily inhabited by quiet old ladies, she was given between 300 and 800 milligrams of Thorazine a day. She was described as "very anxious and fearful" the day she came to Building O and as "very anxious and fearful" the day she left. On August 14, she was moved to Building L, another unpleasant back ward for chronic patients. She came to Building L screaming and was put in the cage room — a room off a corridor near the dayhall that resembled a cage in a zoo. Instead of having bars in front, the cage room had a mesh screen, through which attendants could watch the patients they had confined. The doctor who interviewed Miss Frumkin shortly after her arrival in Building L described her as "agitated, panicky, restless, pacing up and down, handling and touching all objects in her reach, relighting and extinguishing cigarettes." She admitted to him that she had hallucinations. ("Thinks that she might be Christ, the voice of God, etc.") When Joyce Frumkin came to visit her sister in Building L, Sylvia held out her bare hands to show Joyce what she described as her stigmata.

One of the attendants on the day shift in Building L was Evelyn Deacon, the attendant who was known for disliking any patient who, like Sylvia Frumkin, was both "arrogant" and difficult. Miss Frumkin tried to escape whenever a ward door was opened. The doctor in charge of Building L often ordered her put into a straitjacket "for safety of self and others." He once told her parents that the straitjacket made her feel secure. Mrs. Deacon carried out the doctor's orders with enthusiasm. She didn't just put Miss Frumkin into a straitjacket; she also tied a sheet around her shoulders and used it to tie the straitjacketed Miss Frumkin to a bed. Miss Frumkin spent most of September and the first part of October in a straitjacket. She was not allowed to have visitors very often, but once, when her mother came to see her, she said, "Ma, it's not me that's in here, it's the illness. The illness is stronger than I am."

On September 24, after Miss Frumkin had been given assorted small doses of different drugs, she was given 10 milligrams of Haldol. On October 1, her daily dose of Haldol was increased to 15 milligrams (the equivalent of 750 milligrams of Thorazine), and, in addition, she was given 60 milligrams of Valium. Her condition improved in October. As has so often been the case with her, it was not clear whether that particular dose of Haldol and Valium was sufficient at that particular point in her illness to cause her symptoms to subside or whether that particular episode of schizophrenia was finally coming to an end. Whatever the case, she did improve, although the improvement was not detectable in the notes that Mrs. Deacon continued to write about her. On October 12, Mrs. Deacon described Miss Frumkin as "very disrespectful to pts. & employees, tells them she has degrees from Hunter College & more than they have, has to be observed at all times." On November 10: "Very untidy, dislikes to shower & change her clothes, refuses to wash her underwear like the other young patients, she is very pesty."

In November of 1968, Mrs. Poster, the psychiatric social worker in the insulin unit, heard via the Creedmoor grapevine of Miss Frumkin's troubles with Mrs. Deacon. Mrs. Poster set out to do two things: She wanted to help Miss Frumkin get out of the hospital, and at the same time she wanted to keep her from having to return home. There were no halfway houses for Creedmoor patients in Queens at that time, but Mrs. Poster knew of a halfway house for former mental patients called Cobble Hill, which had opened in Brooklyn in 1967. Although the Frumkins were opposed to Sylvia's not living at home, their opposition did not deter Mrs. Poster from proceeding, because she believed that what she was doing was in the patient's interest. She got Miss Frumkin into Cobble Hill.

On January 27, 1969, the psychiatrist in charge of Building L discharged Miss Frumkin from Creedmoor, noting that she was "in a good state of remission with no thought disorders." Her diagnosis was still schizophrenia, undifferentiated type. Her condition was "improved." That same day, Irving Frumkin promised the hospital that he would see to it that Sylvia continued taking her fifteen milligrams a day of Haldol and her Valium, which had been reduced to thirty milligrams a day. Mrs. Deacon's next-to-last note on Miss

Frumkin in early January read, "Patient has very bad manners, table manners included. Patients do not want to sit at the table with her therefore we have to sit her at a table alone." Her last note, on January 27, said simply, "Patient discharged today to Cobble Hill, all clothing and personal property released to Pt."

⸻

The discharge plans for Miss Frumkin, which had taken about two months to make, lasted about two months. When Joyce Frumkin visited Sylvia at Cobble Hill, she found it a decent place. There were a number of group meetings for the residents — living-skills groups, current-events groups, socialization groups. Sylvia had a small private room. Irving Frumkin came to visit her every second day. She would not keep her room clean, and was asked to leave in March. She moved from Cobble Hill to Tatham House, a YWCA residence on Lexington Avenue at Thirty-eighth Street.

Through the efforts of the New York State Division of Vocational Rehabilitation, which had an extensive pre-vocational pilot program at Creedmoor, arrangements were made for Miss Frumkin to attend the Midtown School of Business, in Manhattan, at DVR expense. At Midtown, she studied shorthand, typing, and business English. In October of 1968, just as the Haldol may have begun to help Miss Frumkin, her father had turned against neuroleptics. He had arranged for Dr. Gerald Simmons, a specialist in megavitamins, to visit Sylvia at Creedmoor. After interviewing her, Dr. Simmons had told her and her parents that she would be a good candidate for megavitamins. The doctor in Building L had said that she was doing well on Haldol and Valium, and that he preferred to keep her on just those two drugs for the time being. In the spring of 1969, however, Mr. Frumkin took Sylvia to see Dr. Simmons. She started taking megavitamins.

For several months in the summer and fall of 1969, Miss Frumkin was pleased with Midtown, with megavitamins, and with the Tatham Y. She later looked back on the Tatham YWCA as "the best place I've ever lived," because "it was the closest I ever came to living independently." In the fall, Miss Frumkin decided that the megavitamins weren't agreeing with her, and stopped taking all her medication. She soon dropped out of the Midtown School of Business.

The following month, Harriet Frumkin received a telephone call from the manager of the Tatham Y. He told her that Sylvia's room was absolutely filthy, that Sylvia was riding up and down in the elevator, and that she would have to leave the Y. The Frumkins came to the Tatham Y to fetch Sylvia and her belongings. By the time they got there, she had disappeared. When they packed up her belongings, they noticed that there were no megavitamins in her room. Sylvia had thrown them away, along with the Haldol and Valium she was supposed to be taking. The Frumkins called Dr. Simmons. Sylvia was in his office. She was psychotic. She wanted to go to Gracie Square Hospital, and was admitted there on December 21, 1969. She had been out of Creedmoor for almost eleven months. Studies show that between eighty and ninety percent of the patients who fail to take their neuroleptic medication after the remission of a psychotic episode will have to be rehospitalized within two years, but of the patients who take their medication the percentage that require rehospitalization is reduced by half.

Miss Frumkin went to Gracie Square on December 21, 1969, insisting that she was pregnant with Paul McCartney's baby. She was transferred to St. Vincent's on January 28, 1970, with her delusion intact. She received twenty ECT treatments at St. Vincent's, and has few memories of her stay there. After ninety days, she was released in a fragile condition. She lived at home for a few days, had a bad fight with her mother one evening, and returned to Creedmoor on May 3, 1970.

Sixteen

The Creedmoor to which Miss Frumkin was admitted in May of 1970 was a different hospital from the one she had left in January of 1969. In February of 1969, the new director, Dr. Irwin M. Greenberg, had reorganized the hospital. He transformed the former admissions wards and back wards into geographical units to serve the various sections of Queens. All the patients then at Creedmoor — the "disturbed," the "chronic old ladies," and the newly admitted — were put into the unit that corresponded to the section of Queens in which they had lived before they were hospitalized; thereafter, each unit took new patients from its section of the borough. Each unit was supposed to work with its own community to expedite the release of patients and provide them with treatment after their release. Transitional facilities, known as hotel wards, were opened for patients who didn't need to live in locked wards but were not yet able to return to the community.

Consequently, Sylvia Frumkin was admitted to the geographical unit that encompassed Beechhurst. Although she came in excited, admitted to hearing the voice of her late grandmother, and screamed that her parents were interfering too much in her private life, she wanted to be helped, and signed a voluntary form. Dr. Hans Fogel, the psychiatrist who admitted her, diagnosed her illness as schizophrenia, paranoid type. He started Miss Frumkin on a daily dosage of 1200 milligrams of Thorazine, 30 milligrams of Haldol, and 15 milligrams of Prolixin — the equivalent of 3450 milligrams of Thorazine — and 60 milligrams of Valium. The unit attendants all noted that despite the large dose of drugs Miss Frumkin was getting, there was no improvement in her condition. In June, her medication was 1200 milligrams of Thorazine, 40 milligrams of Stelazine, and 10 milligrams of Haldol — the equivalent of 2500 milligrams of Thorazine — and in addition to this array of neuroleptics she was still getting 60 milligrams of Valium a day. Polypharmacy was rampant in the early 1970s. It was stopped in the late seventies at Creedmoor and at New York State's other mental hospitals, because studies had by then shown it to be a misguided policy. When a patient is taking several neuroleptics at once, one or more may be working and one or more may be causing undesirable side effects, and it is hard to tell which is responsible for what; moreover, the patient is being exposed to the side effects of all the drugs. Polypharmacy is still practiced in many private and voluntary hospitals. In June, Miss Frumkin cried a lot and asked for help; her parents were advised not to visit. In July, the Frumkins talked Dr. Fogel into letting Sylvia take megavitamins. Dr. Fogel didn't believe that they were effective in treating most types of schizophrenia, but he thought they would not harm her as long as she continued to take neuroleptics. According to a study of neuroleptics and megavitamins that was later done on hospitalized schizophrenic patients, those who were given megavitamins as well as neuroleptics not only had to stay in the hospital longer but also needed larger doses of the neuroleptics than those who received neuroleptics alone. The reason for the difference is unknown. In late July, Miss Frumkin's condition nevertheless started to improve. Her parents were able to visit, and she was able to go out with them on weekends and to go on home visits. Dr. Fogel thought it might be beneficial for her to do some typing in his office. She was pleased to type for him, and the attendants' notes show that in August and early September she became friendlier, more cooperative, and more sociable. Her medication was gradually lowered.

In September of 1970, Miss Frumkin was admitted to a hotel ward and began a nurse's-aide training program in Building 40. She did well in the nurse's-aide program. A few weeks later, she tried to commit suicide by swallowing a bottle of Stelazine tablets, and was rushed to Flushing Hospital to have her stomach pumped. On November 15, 1970, Miss Frumkin was released from Creedmoor on "convalescent care." She went home to live, and completed the nurse's-aide program in December as an out-patient. She was to continue taking 10 milligrams of Haldol and 40 milligrams of Stelazine — the equivalent of 1300 milligrams of Thorazine.

In December of 1970, shortly after completing the nurse's-aide program, Miss Frumkin went out to look for a job. She had heard that a nurse's-aide position was available in a nursing home only a few minutes away from the Frumkins' house. She went there with a résumé she had typed up. The woman who interviewed her noticed that there was nothing between her graduation from high school, in June of 1966, and December of 1970, except three months at the Midtown School of Business, and asked her why. Miss Frumkin told the woman that she had been a patient at Creedmoor a good deal of that time and had just graduated from a nurse's-aide program given at Creedmoor. The nurse's-aide position evaporated. Miss Frumkin came home from the interview feeling dejected. She stayed at home for several weeks, sleeping most of the time. She was too dazed to seek another job as a nurse's aide. A friend of her mother's was the executive secretary of a national charitable organization. She felt sorry for Sylvia and offered her a job there as a clerical assistant.

Three months later, another of Harriet Frumkin's friends, who worked at Long Island Jewish Medical Center, helped get Sylvia into a vocational-rehabilitation program there. Between April and September of 1971, she worked as a clerical assistant in the L.I.J. Adolescent Clinic. As a result of her capable performance there, the Division of Vocational Rehabilitation placed her at the Mandl School for Medical and Dental Assistants, in midtown Manhattan. Sylvia Frumkin wanted to become a medical assistant, but when she was tested at Mandl she was found to be too uncoordinated to do the lab work that was part of the medical-assistant course. She was advised to take the medical-secretary course instead. Dr. Fogel, whom Miss Frumkin had continued to see once a week, as a private patient, since her release from Creedmoor, also advised her to take that course, because he thought it would be less stressful. Both courses lasted ten months, but the medical-assistant course was in session for six or seven hours a day, while the medical-secretary course was in session for four or five hours. Among the subjects that Miss Frumkin studied at the Mandl School were medical terminology and usage, medical typing, and medical stenography and transcription.

The ten months between September of 1971, when Miss Frumkin started at Mandl, and July of 1972, when she satisfactorily completed the medical-secretary course and earned a certificate from the Mandl School, were the ten best months she had had since January of 1964, when she was hit by the car. It was the first time since 1966, when she was a senior in high school, that she had had real hope for the future. She was glad to be back at school during the week, with a group of "normal" young women; she was the only student in the class who was subsidized by the DVR, and she kept that fact to herself. She liked the curriculum at Mandl, and she liked wearing the required white uniform and white shoes. On Saturdays, she worked as a receptionist in the Bronx office of the Frumkins' internist, who paid her ten dollars per Saturday. He had hired her as a favor, but he was satisfied with her work. She was well liked by his patients.

When Miss Frumkin was discharged from Creedmoor in 1969, she weighed 175 pounds. When she was discharged from Creedmoor in 1970, she weighed 180 pounds. In the fall of 1971, she decided to go to Weight Watchers. She was told that the ideal weight for her height and build was 132. She stuck to the Weight Watchers precise diet faithfully and lost weight consistently. She loved going to the weekly Weight Watchers meetings to get on the scale. All those present who had lost weight were applauded. She received applause almost every week. Her weight went down to 119 — less than it had been when she was fourteen. She lightened her hair with a blond spray and bought some pretty new clothes. Most of them were size 9, 10, or 11 but she was especially proud of one uniform, which was size 8.

While Miss Frumkin was in Creedmoor in 1970, she had met a young man named John Yarrow. Yarrow had been hospitalized for six weeks in 1970 after taking an overdose of diet pills; since his release, he had worked as a postal clerk. Every payday, he telephoned Miss Frumkin and asked her where she wanted to go on Saturday night. He took her to restaurants, to movies, to Gilbert and Sullivan operettas, and to plays. John Yarrow's parents owned a pharmacy. Harriet and Irving Frumkin thought that John Yarrow was a "real gentleman," and hoped that Sylvia would marry him. Sylvia liked the places to which John took her, but she was indifferent to John himself. She considered him a mama's boy and thought him less intelligent and less artistic than she was. She also looked down on him because at a time when she was newly slender and quite attractive he was very fat and homely. He had brown stains on his teeth from smoking cigarettes, and green lips from chewing Clorets. He perspired profusely in the heat, and she disliked his body odor. Sylvia told Joyce that she couldn't stand the way he kissed her and that he didn't know how to make love. While Sylvia was going out with John, she was also seeing Stanley Gordon, a former sixth-grade classmate who had just returned from a Midwestern university with a Ph.D. in anthropology. One day, he told her that he loved her but that he wasn't in love with her and didn't feel physically attracted to her. She felt injured, because she had just worked so hard to make herself physically attractive. Joyce fixed her up with a blind date, and so did one of her cousins. Both of the blind dates were handsome men. She liked them and hoped they would ask her out again, but they didn't. "The ones that liked me I didn't like," Miss Frumkin says. "The ones I liked didn't like me."

In the spring of 1972, Miss Frumkin stopped going out with John Yarrow. She stopped going to Weight Watchers, and within two months she weighed 147 pounds. "Once there was no more applause, I started to eat," she said recently. "When I was thin, I bought myself an ordinary two-piece bathing suit rather than a bikini, because I knew that somehow I'd gain the weight back." Instead of going to Weight Watchers, she went to Buddhist meetings. One afternoon on her way home from the Mandl School, she had met a woman named Daisy Hayes. Mrs. Hayes and her husband, Mark, were the leaders of a Buddhist group. At her first Buddhist meeting, Sylvia met a young man, left the meeting with him, and went to his apartment. They made love. Years later, she recalled the Buddhist as "the only guy I ever enjoyed sex with." He discarded her after two days, but she continued to go to Buddhist meetings, and she chanted mantras at home. That spring, she was assigned a term project by the Mandl School. As her project, she chose to compile a dictionary of medical definitions. It was due in mid-June. Term papers at Music and Art and at the high school in Queens had always frightened her, because they were long and she was afraid she wouldn't finish them on time. She became so nervous about her medical dictionary that Dr.

Fogel lent her one of his costly medical reference works and prescribed Tofranil, a tricyclic antidepressant drug, for her. Before she started her medical dictionary, she had been busily making plans for the future. After her graduation ceremony from the Mandl School, which was to be held on July 10, she was going to get a full-time job working for a friend of the internist. She was going to refurnish her room. She hoped to go on a vacation. In June, she became increasingly nervous. The Tofranil seemed to be making her worse instead of better, so she stopped taking all her medication. (For reasons that are still unclear, when tricyclic antidepressants are given to some schizophrenics, either alone or in conjunction with neuroleptics, they may activate a psychosis.) Miss Frumkin suddenly got tired of Dr. Fogel and stopped seeing him. The internist for whom she was working recommended a psychologist to her. She handed in her medical dictionary two weeks late. She got it back marked A+ shortly before she was to graduate.

On the evening of July 9, Miss Frumkin started burning incense in her room and chanting to Buddha. She was wearing a red velours robe with gold trim that she referred to as her monk's robe. She ran out of the house. Two days later, the Frumkins learned that she had been admitted to Elmhurst, a municipal hospital in Queens. While Sylvia was missing on July 10, Mrs. Frumkin went to the Mandl School's graduation ceremony to get her daughter's medical-secretary certificate; she told the school officials that Sylvia was at home with a fever. She had tried to talk her husband into accompanying her. "If you want to be a masochist, go," Mr. Frumkin had said. He had stayed home. The twenty months from November of 1970 to July of 1972 was the longest period that Miss Frumkin was out of a hospital between 1964 (when she was first admitted to Gracie Square) and 1981. To this day, Mrs. Frumkin looks back on Sylvia's ten months at the Mandl School wistfully. "It was the most normal Sylvia has been since she was a child," she says.

IV

The Air Is Too Still

Seventeen

On October 25, 1972, on the certification of two physicians (or two P.C.), Sylvia Frumkin was transferred to Creedmoor and placed in the unit that handled patients from Beechhurst: the Clearview unit. At that time, part of the Clearview unit occupied two floors of an eyesore known as Building 25. Miss Frumkin was in an agitated, restless, and anxious condition; she was overtalkative, and was found to be lacking in insight and judgment. A doctor who gave her a mental examination the day after her admission recorded the way her mind was running the events of her recent past through its kaleidoscope:

> (Why here?) I'm finding Sylvia and I think it's lovely to stay with beautiful people. (Problem) I graduated from a secretarial school but I didn't go to work. (Why?) My mother is mothering me too much. I got away besides the nicotine gets into my sputum and makes me nervous. This is the reason why I play rock music and the guitar. (What do you do at home?) I listen to the radio but I kept on thinking that I need a blood test and a pap smear. (Did you have any contact?) Maybe. (Ideas of harming yourself?) I was foolish to take all my pills once but I immediately woke my parents. (Why do you get angry?) I twisted my mother's arm before I came here.

For about a week, Miss Frumkin stopped smoking, kept herself neat, and took her medication. She told a therapy aide that she liked Creedmoor, "because I always get well here" — something she often said ten minutes after saying that Creedmoor was hell. By early November, the therapy aides were noting that Miss Frumkin was uncooperative and untidy, threatened them with lawsuits, wore bizarre clothes, chain-smoked, and disturbed other patients in the dormitory by sitting on the floor all night praying. At the end of November, a nurse noted that Miss Frumkin pretended to take her medication but was caught throwing it into a garbage can. At the beginning of December, a nurse noted that she enjoyed foraging through the garbage cans and that she often sought out secluded areas with male patients.

On December 24, 1972, when her two P.C. expired, Miss Frumkin signed a voluntary form agreeing to remain at Creedmoor. On January 9, 1973, an attendant on the 4:00-to-12:30 shift noticed around suppertime that Miss Frumkin was missing. The attendant telephoned the Frumkins. Sylvia wasn't at home. The following day, the Frumkins received a call from Daisy and Mark Hayes, who had heard from Sylvia. She was at LaGuardia Airport. She had left the hospital with another patient, a young man named Jean-Paul. They had decided to stow away on a plane and go to California. An airline ticket agent had become suspicious of Sylvia and Jean-Paul when Sylvia had addressed the agent as Peter Sellers. Jean-Paul had sensed the agent's suspicion and had fled, leaving Sylvia alone at the airport with her fantasy that she was going to Hollywood to make a movie and that all the people she met along the way were in the movie with her. She had telephoned the Hayeses, had told them where she was, and had said that she wanted to go either to California or to their house. The Hayeses had then telephoned the Frumkins. Sylvia's father, Irving Frumkin, went to LaGuardia with the Hayeses while Harriet Frumkin telephoned Creedmoor to tell the attendants on duty at Clearview where Sylvia was. Three Clearview attendants went to LaGuardia and took her back to the ward. After her return to the hospital, her medication was increased slightly. In January and early February, according to her medical records, she still spent a good deal of her time pursuing young men "in a very unladylike manner, letting them feel her and she them, kissing openly in public." (Irving and Harriet Frumkin had much preferred the sexual segregation that existed until 1969.) Miss Frumkin had been given moderate doses of four neuroleptics during the fall of 1972; when she was given the equivalent of 900 milligrams of Thorazine daily, in January of 1973, her condition improved. Her medication was then inexplicably lowered to the equivalent of 400 milligrams of Thorazine daily, and she was discharged on March 20, 1973. She was to live at home and go to the Clearview Day Center on weekdays as an out-patient.

Miss Frumkin went to the Day Center a few times, and then began going to Buddhist meetings instead. While she was attending medical-secretary school, she had planned to refurnish her room, but she had never done so. In 1973, she no longer even wanted her old furniture; she wanted to convert her room into a Buddhist shrine, with wall-to-wall pillows and prayer rugs. Mrs. Frumkin refused to throw any furniture out, but she occasionally tried to pacify Sylvia by ringing gongs with her. One evening in April, Sylvia didn't return home. At a Buddhist meeting she had attended that afternoon, the guest speaker was a man named Daniel Eiseman, who ran a halfway house for former mental patients on the fourteenth floor of the Hotel Martinique, on West Thirty-second Street near Greeley Square, in Manhattan. Eiseman was a Buddhist, a social worker, and a proponent of megavitamins. The residents of his halfway house received megavitamins from a doctor affiliated with a nearby clinic that specialized in them. The day after the Buddhist meeting, Eiseman called the Frumkins, introduced himself, and said, "If your daughter is Sylvia Frumkin, she's with us, she's safe, and she's getting megavitamins."

The Frumkins went to the Hotel Martinique to visit Sylvia

and to drop off some of her belongings — clothes, cosmetics, records. She seemed content there. The Martinique had once been a thriving commercial hotel (it was in the garment district), but by 1973 it had fallen on hard times. It was one of many hotels in midtown and on upper Broadway that had become single-room-occupancy hotels, or SROs, filled with welfare clients and former mental patients. SROs and adult homes proliferated after the Department of Mental Hygiene decided to depopulate the state hospitals. In fact, many critics said that, for the sake of accuracy, the department's policy should be called not deinstitutionalization but trans-institutionalization. The new institutions were not limited to the SROs and adult homes, many of which housed former patients in conditions even more tawdry than those prevailing in the state hospitals. There were also so-called skilled-nursing facilities, or SNFs, and health-related facilities, or HRFs. Many former patients simply wound up as derelicts. As late as 1980, eighty percent of the New York State mental-health budget still went to the depopulated state hospitals; the public had accepted the idea of community mental-health care as long as the community mental-health-care facilities were situated in someone else's community.

One evening in June of 1973, Miss Frumkin went to a bar with another resident of the halfway house and got drunk. She returned to the Hotel Martinique, where she faintly remembers dancing around the fourteenth floor in a nightgown she had ornamented with jujubes. She then grabbed an armful of records, went downstairs, and started dancing around in Greeley Square, giving out records to a crowd that quickly assembled. Eiseman telephoned the Frumkins. He told Mrs. Frumkin that Sylvia had gone berserk, and that she would have to come and get her daughter, because he couldn't handle her anymore. Mr. Frumkin was out. Mrs. Frumkin took the subway into the city. When she got to Greeley Square, she saw a large crowd. "Look at that crazy girl," a woman standing next to Mrs. Frumkin said, pointing to a young woman who was dressed only in a bra and a half-slip as she danced and distributed records. Mrs. Frumkin recognized Sylvia. "You should be thankful it's not your daughter," she said to the woman. Then two policemen arrived. One of them covered Miss Frumkin with his jacket, and they took her to Bellevue. She remained there several weeks. She was given high doses of Thorazine during the first part of her stay and no medication at all during the latter part, but neither form of treatment kept her from believing that, as a result of her chanting, both Queen Elizabeth and President Nixon had come to visit her. On July 16, she was transferred to Creedmoor on a two P.C.

When the doctor in the Clearview unit who had discharged Sylvia Frumkin on March 20 learned that she was back, he remarked to a colleague that in the pre-neuroleptic era she would have been permanently confined to Creedmoor. The drugs had made it possible for her to be a mobile chronic schizophrenic. He predicted that she would spend the next twenty years in and out of hospitals. What he didn't predict was just how often she would be in and out of Creedmoor in the six months following her fifth admission to the hospital. On July 22, she escaped. On July 31, the police picked her up on the street and took her to Elmhurst. She has never been disposed to reveal where she was during those nine days. On August 28, after she had spent four weeks at Elmhurst walking around naked, spitting out her medication, and hitting a number of patients and attendants, Elmhurst sent her back to Creedmoor. She next escaped from Creedmoor on September 8, and she resurfaced at Manhattan Psychiatric Hospital, on Wards Island, on September 10. Manhattan Psychiatric's plan was to send Miss Frumkin back to Creedmoor, but Miss Frumkin had another plan. She walked out of the hospital, hailed a taxi, and rode home. Her parents took her back to Creedmoor that same day, with the assistance of one of their friends. On September 26, Miss Frumkin asked to go to Jewish services. She was given permission to go, under the supervision of a male therapy aide. After the services, while refreshments were being served, she slipped away from the therapy aide. She arrived home that evening. Before her parents could calm her down or telephone Creedmoor, she cut the telephone line with a pair of scissors, said that she didn't want to go back to Creedmoor, and ran out of the house. A few hours later, two patrolmen picked her up on the Throgs Neck Bridge, not far away. She was still carrying the pair of scissors, and was aggressive and abusive. The policemen took her back to Creedmoor. On September 18, when the two P.C. had expired, Dr. William L. Werner, who had taken over as Creedmoor's director in 1972, had applied for a court order of retention, because the psychiatrists in the Clearview unit believed that Miss Frumkin was not well enough to be discharged. On October 23, 1973, Miss Frumkin and a court-appointed lawyer appeared at a hearing, in Creedmoor's Building 40, before a judge of the New York State Supreme Court for Queens County. The judge ordered that Miss Frumkin be retained for a period not to exceed six months. She decided to exercise her right to petition the court for a rehearing. The court-appointed lawyer represented Miss Frumkin at the rehearing, and, in addition, the court designated an independent psychiatrist to examine her. A psychiatrist on the Clearview staff described her at this time as "dysfunctional even within the hospital environment." The court-appointed psychiatrist interviewed her and concluded that she should not be discharged. On December 19, a Supreme Court judge and six jurors met and decided that Miss Frumkin should be continued on her present court commitment. She tried to escape as she was returning to Building 25, but she was restrained.

Whenever Miss Frumkin had not been absent without leave from Creedmoor between July and December, she had been receiving moderate doses of various neuroleptics, which didn't have any effect on her. She had tried to pull off the wigs that some of the female therapy aides wore, had changed her clothes ten times before she could be persuaded to leave the dormitory in the morning, had fought with female patients, and had had sex with male patients. Her medication was changed often, and she often demanded to see the medication cards accompanying her medication cups. On the morning of January 27, 1974, a therapy aide named Mary Dodd was giving out medication in Miss Frumkin's ward. When Mrs. Dodd handed Miss Frumkin her pills, she accused Mrs. Dodd of giving her the wrong medication. Mrs. Dodd told her she was simply giving her what the doctor had ordered. Miss Frumkin started screaming at Mrs. Dodd. When Mrs. Dodd tried to pour water into Miss Frumkin's medication cup, Miss Frumkin spit the pills at Mrs. Dodd and spilled water all over Mrs. Dodd and herself. Another patient assisted Mrs. Dodd by taking the medication tray. Miss Frumkin hit Mrs. Dodd. "I finally remembered that if anyone is having hysterics, a slap calms them; so I slapped her on the face, not in anger or to harm her but to calm her, which it did," Mrs. Dodd later reported. Mrs. Dodd was brought up on disciplinary charges, because at Creedmoor hitting a patient is forbidden, no matter what the provocation. After statements were taken from Miss Frumkin (whose account of the event varied each time she was questioned), from Mrs. Dodd, and from the patient who had assisted her, Mrs. Dodd was first given an official reprimand. She contested the reprimand, which the hospital eventually agreed to withdraw, for several reasons: Mrs. Dodd had worked at Creedmoor for nearly four years and had never done anything that required special counseling or disciplinary action; Miss Frumkin was the source of a good deal of conflict in the ward, because she frequently provoked attacks on herself, then greatly exaggerated or completely fantasized the behavior of others in these incidents; and in the opinion of her supervisor, Mrs. Dodd's explanation of why she had hit Miss Frumkin indicated "scrupulous honesty as well as the need for training in the management of disturbed patients." Instead of the reprimand, Mrs. Dodd was given some training in the management of disturbed, assaultive patients. She worked at Creedmoor until her death, in 1980, and was never again brought up on disciplinary charges.

On January 19, 1974, Miss Frumkin's medication had been changed to 80 milligrams of Stelazine daily — the equivalent of 1600 milligrams of Thorazine, and a higher dose than the total of the potpourri of drugs she had previously received. In late February, her condition took a turn for the better. Her personal appearance and behavior continued to improve in March. She started going home on visits and went to a typing program on the Creedmoor grounds several times.

In March of 1974, Harriet and Irving Frumkin met with the Clearview social worker to discuss Sylvia's discharge. The Frumkins had by then become active in the Long Island Schizophrenia Association. One member of LISA had given them a pamphlet about Gould Farm, a community rehabilitation center that occupied six hundred acres in the Berkshires, in western Massachusetts. Gould Farm's community was composed of about thirty full-time staff members, their spouses and children, and about forty guests — both men and women, most of them between the ages of nineteen and forty. Many of the guests had been in psychiatric hospitals, but Gould Farm accepted only people who were "in a reasonably good state of remission." The brochure made it clear that Gould Farm could not offer anyone a permanent home; most guests stayed for a period of between three months and a year. In early April, Miss Frumkin was given a week's leave from Creedmoor. The Frumkins had made an appointment at Gould Farm, and they drove Sylvia there for a required twenty-four-hour trial visit. They liked Gould Farm immediately. Sylvia was accepted there. The Frumkins drove her back to New York. She returned to Creedmoor for a few days, had the court order dropped, and was discharged.

⸗ ⸗ ⸗

There were two residential buildings at Gould Farm, each supervised by houseparents. Guests had private rooms, and were required to take care of their rooms and their personal hygiene. They were also required to work six hours a day, helping in the dining room, in the kitchen, or on a hundred acres that were used for farming. Gould Farm raised most of its own meat and vegetables. Its dairy herd provided the farm with all its milk, its flock of chickens provided eggs. Chores were rotated. Miss Frumkin gathered eggs, set tables, and did her share of the seasonal chores — raking leaves, shoveling snow, clearing trails, making maple syrup. The guests had the rest of the day free to go to square dances, parties, and community meetings; to take trips to movies and concerts; to engage in sports; or to spend time in the weaving studio and the craft shop. At Gould Farm, Miss Frumkin learned to weave, to do needlepoint, and to crochet.

The first thing Miss Frumkin did at Gould Farm was to give up smoking — a habit with which she had always felt uneasy. The second thing she did was to start gaining weight on the ample breakfasts, lunches, dinners, midmorning coffee breaks, afternoon teas, and bedtime snacks provided. She was also caught skimming cream off the tops of bottles of unhomogenized milk in the milk room. After several months at Gould Farm, she weighed 196 pounds. She decided to go to a Weight Watchers group in the nearby town of Great Barrington. The executive director of Gould Farm remembers her running compulsively from table to table snatching meat from other guests' plates, to be sure of having precisely the number of ounces of chicken or liver specified in the Weight Watchers diet; he came to regret having given his approval to her going to Weight Watchers. She lost some weight, but she did not stick with Weight Watchers long; diets lost their charm for Sylvia Frumkin as quickly as psychiatrists did.

During her first months at Gould Farm, Miss Frumkin was still taking eighty milligrams of Stelazine a day, which she had been advised to do when she left Creedmoor, along with six milligrams of Cogentin and some Dalmane (she had had some trouble sleeping). She was also taking megavitamins.

Gould Farm had a consulting psychiatrist, Dr. Dale Greaney, who came to the farm once a week to see the guests. A few months after Sylvia's arrival, Dr. Greaney began to see her every second or third week for between half an hour and forty-five minutes. Sylvia was always lucid but circuitous. In Dr. Greaney's opinion, she was no more and no less ill than most of the other chronic-schizophrenic guests he saw at Gould Farm, but three things did set her apart from the others. The first was her physical clumsiness and lack of coordination. Like several other psychiatrists who have treated Miss Frumkin, Dr. Greaney believed that she might have a neurological problem. He sent her to a neurologist for a consultation. The neurologist gave her a thorough examination and a test to rule out the possibility that she might have Wilson's disease, a hereditary condition characterized by toxic deposits of copper in many organs and tissues, including the central nervous system; the test was negative. The neurologist also determined that she didn't have any other neurological problem that would explain her behavior. (As a consequence of the neurologist's examination, Miss Frumkin came to believe that she did have Wilson's disease, just as insulin-coma therapy, which she had had in 1967, had convinced her that she suffered from hypoglycemia.) The second thing that made her different from guests at Gould Farm with whom she shared many of the symptoms of schizophrenia was her imperious behavior. Dr. Greaney knew many schizophrenics who were quiet, were neat and kept their rooms clean, and had good manners. Miss Frumkin was loud, her room was messy, and she irritated most people at Gould Farm by her social clumsiness. She grated on her fellow-guests and on the staff by literally and figuratively stepping on their toes; she seemed to lack any sense of where she ended and the next person began. The third thing that he believed set Miss Frumkin apart from other schizophrenics he had seen was her unwillingness to settle for the half life of halfway houses and "sheltered workshops," as so many chronic schizophrenics did.

Some months after Miss Frumkin began to see Dr. Greaney, her legs started to move back and forth involuntarily when she was seated. He changed her medication from 80 milligrams of Stelazine to 600 milligrams of Mellaril, which was the equivalent of 600 milligrams of Thorazine — a reduction of over sixty percent in her medication. When Dr. Greaney had gone into private practice, in 1973, he had been antagonistic to medication. He had hoped to treat schizophrenic patients without drugs. Experience had taught him that he couldn't, but he continued to prefer talking to people (his main interest now is couples therapy) rather than medicating them. Eventually, he relinquished part of his job at Gould Farm to another psychiatrist, one reason being that "the work was almost all writing prescriptions." He now goes to Gould Farm half a day a week. Dr. Greaney changed Miss Frumkin's medication from Stelazine to Mellaril because he believed that of all the neuroleptics Mellaril caused the least hyperactivity. In choosing Mellaril (there were alternative ways to deal with the leg swinging), he chose one of the few drugs that could not be safely given in a dose comparable to 80 milligrams of Stelazine. Mellaril, unlike most neuroleptics, has an absolute ceiling — 800 milligrams. The manufacturer warns that higher doses can cause pigmentary retinopathy — a discoloration of the retina that impairs vision. Dr. Greaney didn't worry about decreasing Miss Frumkin's medication, and didn't even give her the maximum dosage of Mellaril. He regularly reduced the medication of guests at Gould Farm by anywhere from twenty-five to fifty percent, because the guests worked six hours a day and he observed that they became too tired if they took the same medication they had been given while they were leading inactive lives in hospitals. He didn't notice any change in Miss Frumkin's behavior for several months after he lowered her medication. (Some patients "decompensate" twenty-four hours after a reduction or cessation of their neuroleptic medication, and some decompensate only after eighteen months, but the average time is about three months.) Dr. Greaney did notice that Miss Frumkin was suddenly talking a great deal about religion. He decided that her preoccupation with religion was nondelusional and therefore didn't do anything about it.

After Miss Frumkin had been at Gould Farm a year, the staff met with the director to discuss her future. Most guests either suffered relapses and went back to hospitals or improved sufficiently to go to a halfway house or return home. An occasional guest was allowed to stay on at Gould Farm if he or she was no trouble and fitted into the farm's therapeutic community. The staff told the director that no exception should be made for Miss Frumkin. They had hoped that they could change her behavior, and had expended a great deal of energy on her, but she was as obnoxious as she had been when she arrived. On June 1, 1975, Miss Frumkin was told that she would have to leave Gould Farm in three months. The Frumkins were distressed. "Gould Farm was such a wonderful time for us," Harriet Frumkin recalled some years later. "Sylvia was in reasonably good shape, she wasn't in a hospital, and she was *away*." The Frumkins knew from having had Sylvia living at home several times in the early 1970s that it would be better for the whole family if she did not return there. The social worker at Gould Farm tried to get her into a number of halfway houses in Massachusetts, where she had placed other Gould Farm guests. Miss Frumkin was unenthusiastic about the halfway houses, and they were unenthusiastic about her. Between June and September, as she was threatened with the sort of change that had triggered psychotic episodes in the past, and was more vulnerable because her medication had been lowered, she began to decompensate more visibly. She became increasingly preoccupied with religion. Unknown to some people at Gould Farm, Miss Frumkin had met a member of the American Board of Missions to the Jews one Saturday in 1972 on her way home from the internist's office where she was then working. Members of the ABMJ are primarily Jews who believe that Jesus is the Messiah; they consider themselves spiritually reborn, and believe that their purpose in life is to bring the message of Jesus to other Jews. Miss Frumkin had not pursued the invitation to become converted to Christianity in 1972; instead, she had become a Buddhist in 1973. She had turned against the Buddhists after she was asked to leave the Hotel Martinique. At Creedmoor, after she ran away from Jewish services she had had several counseling sessions with Creedmoor's rabbi, and had once again seemed to accept Judaism. At Gould Farm, however, a guest who was a born-again Christian had converted her to Christianity. She considered herself born again and started to go to church. Although Gould Farm was nonsectarian, its director was an ordained Presbyterian minister, and a few of the staff members were evangelical Christians. As Miss Frumkin became obsessed with Christianity in the summer of 1975, two staff members at Gould Farm were counseled against proselytizing her. As the deadline for leaving approached, her room became "a disgrace," she stopped taking her medication, and she started running around without any clothes on. The director telephoned the Frumkins and told them they would have to come and get their daughter.

Dr. Greaney was on vacation on August 29, when Miss Frumkin left Gould Farm; he was not surprised to learn later that her exit had been a dramatic one. He recognized that even though her ability to function had become increasingly impaired as she had grown older, her will to succeed had survived. The reason that the staff at Gould Farm felt that her prognosis was so poor was that they could not imagine an entry point into any normal life for Miss Frumkin. At staff meetings, they asked each other, "What would she do?" She couldn't even be hired as a clerk, because of the awkward way in which she presented herself, and, on top of that, she didn't really want to be a clerk. She still wanted to be a star. Dr. Greaney believed that Miss Frumkin's combination of intelligence and grandiosity not only made her prognosis poor but also accounted for the Dionysian quality of her psychotic episodes. "If you have to be Sylvia Frumkin, maybe this is the way to be," he said not long ago. "Many schizophrenics are grandiose, but she has such a high intelligence coupled with her grandiosity. If you see yourself going from defeat to defeat, and the next awesome chasm presents itself and you can't cross it, maybe you stick with the grandiosity in your head instead of facing up to your homeliness and awkwardness and limitations. I think she's a genius at being insane."

⸙ ⸙ ⸙

For two days after her return home, Sylvia fought with her mother. One afternoon, she tossed some of her clothes and books into a small suitcase and ran out of the house. Several hours later, one of the Frumkins' neighbors happened to see her walking on the grass adjacent to the Cross Island Parkway, opening and closing her suitcase as she walked. He brought her home in his car. When she got there, Harriet Frumkin opened the suitcase. Sylvia's clothes and books were gone. In the suitcase were aluminum cans, cigarette butts, and pieces of old tires. Sylvia said she was "helping to clean up the ecology," because it was such a mess. When Mrs. Frumkin shouted at her daughter for losing her clothes and books, Sylvia ran out of the house again. The police found her on a nearby street and took her to Elmhurst. The Frumkins were told that Elmhurst was overcrowded; the hospital could keep her for only a few days before transferring her to Creedmoor.

Sylvia Frumkin didn't want to return to Creedmoor. She got down on her hands and knees and begged her parents not to send her back there. At one of many mental-health meetings that Mr. Frumkin had attended, he had heard of a man named Kenneth Wentworth, a celebrated practitioner of megavitamin therapy. Dr. Wentworth, the director of a clinic in Nassau County, took his private patients to Brunswick Psychiatric Hospital, in Amityville, New York. Sylvia's insurance would cover most of the cost of up to ninety days at Brunswick, but the Frumkins would still have to pay about four hundred dollars a month. Irving Frumkin was willing to send Sylvia to Brunswick. Although there was no proof that megavitamins had ever helped his daughter in the past, he clung to the belief that at Brunswick the megavitamins would be a panacea. Harriet Frumkin was willing, too, after Sylvia put her head in her lap and cried. Joyce Frumkin was opposed to Sylvia's going to Brunswick, and told her parents so. For years, Joyce had been sympathetic to Sylvia. She herself had had a successful career in the fashion industry, going from one well-paid and challenging executive position to another, but she had had a series of unhappy love affairs and had been to a number of therapists in the hope of working out her problems. She and the various therapists attributed many of Joyce's troubles to her family environment. Joyce was especially inclined to blame her father, for putting terrible pressure on her as a child to do well in school and in everything else, but at least one of her therapists believed that while Mr. Frumkin had a bad bark, Mrs. Frumkin had a much worse bite. Joyce believed that she had got off more lightly than Sylvia because she had different genes, but she realized that she had not escaped. She wished she could be happier with herself. She wanted a good marriage and children. For years, whenever Sylvia was in a state of remission Joyce had tried to do the things she thought sisters should do for each other — she had fixed Sylvia up with blind dates, for instance — but by 1975 she had given up on the existence of a cure for Sylvia, and on the possibility of having a sister she could turn to when she was in trouble. Joyce believed that her parents were sending Sylvia to Brunswick because it was better for them to see her in a beautiful hospital than in an ugly one, that they were deluding themselves with false hopes, and that they were throwing good money after bad.

Dr. Wentworth put Miss Frumkin on a special diet, and she lost weight at Brunswick, but though she was receiving neuroleptics and electroshock therapy as well as megavitamins, there was no more than a minor improvement in her condition during her stay there. She was depressed and cried a lot, and she was obsessed with being born again. While she was at Brunswick, Irving Frumkin felt terrible pains in his stomach one evening. He was rushed to the hospital and was operated on for bleeding ulcers.

As Miss Frumkin's ninety days at Brunswick were drawing to an end, her social worker talked to her about her discharge. He thought that an adult home would be the appropriate place for her. The Frumkins drove her to see an adult home called Rockaway Manor. It struck her as a far more horrifying place than Creedmoor. "You expect a state hospital to be awful, but you expect to be treated like a human being in the outside world," she said after seeing the lobby of Rockaway Manor. Mr. Frumkin wanted to place his daughter in the Richmond Fellowship, a transitional-housing program with an excellent reputation, but it had a long waiting list. While Miss Frumkin was still at Brunswick, she telephoned the Manhattan office of the American Board of Missions to the Jews. She spoke of her plight to a man named Alan Goldsmith, and he called George Klopfer, who was in charge of the ABMJ office in Queens. Klopfer went to Brunswick to meet Miss Frumkin, and arrived when her parents were also visiting her. He was appalled at the way she abused them: She seemed to him to be half animal and half human when she yelled at them. He ordered her to quiet down, and she did quiet down. Mr. Frumkin was pale and gaunt after his operation. George Klopfer believed that Sylvia would cause her father's death if she went home with him. Klopfer and his wife, Nellie, lived in a building that the ABMJ owned in Hollis, Queens. Two floors of the house were used for Bible classes and offices; the Klopfers lived on the third floor with a grown son and two young daughters. The Klopfers offered to let Sylvia live with them. Like Benjamin Wilder, they thought that what she needed was a structured environment, which they could provide. Unlike Benjamin Wilder, they believed that Sylvia was possessed by demons — a view of mental illness that was more prevalent in the fifteenth century than in the twentieth. The Klopfers knew that there would be tremendous battles with Sylvia, but they were convinced that they would prevail. Nellie Klopfer had been a registered nurse, and the Klopfers had had some experience with the mentally ill. The Klopfers told the Frumkins that Sylvia, who had studied art as a teenager, could teach their daughters to draw in exchange for her room and board. They agreed to give her megavitamins, although they did not believe in vitamins or any kind of drugs. They believed in the power of Jesus Christ to overcome the forces of Satan.

For a week or two in December, right after Sylvia moved in with them, the Klopfers thought that their way of treating her was effective. Sylvia mumbled a lot. Whenever she mumbled, George Klopfer would intone, "Sylvia, I come against these forces that are making you mumble in the name of Jesus, and I demand by the blood of the lamb that you stop mumbling." Then she would speak clearly. Sylvia was also lazy. She wouldn't clean her room; some days, she wouldn't get out of bed. On her lazy days, Klopfer would recite, "There is power, there is power, there is wonder-working power in the blood of the lamb, in the precious blood of the lamb. I come against these forces in the name of Jesus, and I demand by the blood of the lamb that you dress yourself now. Lord God, we come against these symptoms." Sylvia wouldn't budge.

Sylvia often defied the Klopfers. They told her to read the Gospels of the New Testament; she read the Book of Daniel. They told her to play gospel music on the radio; she played the Top Ten. She was unable by now to draw, much less give drawing lessons. The Klopfers fought relentlessly with Sylvia, believing that her will had to be broken. They were soon battle-weary. She stayed up late, and they got little sleep. They developed sinus headaches. One morning right before Christmas, the Klopfers sat at the breakfast table and prayed that God would eliminate Sylvia from their midst, because they could no longer carry on the struggle. They believed that she was wearing them down as a family. George Klopfer called the Frumkins that evening to say that they had tried their best and failed, and that he was going to take Sylvia to Creedmoor. The Frumkins told him they would meet him there. Sylvia, who had been carrying on at the Klopfers, quieted down as soon as she entered the building that handled nighttime admissions. When the resident on duty screened her, she spoke softly and sensibly. As Klopfer and Harriet and Irving Frumkin all remember it, Sylvia put on a performance worthy of Sarah Bernhardt. "The resident gave us a lecture that made us feel we were monsters to want to put a healthy young woman in a mental hospital," Klopfer recalls. He told the Frumkins that he and Nellie would try again, and he drove Sylvia back to Hollis. Right after New Year's, the Klopfers went with Sylvia to a store in Flushing that was having a going-out-of-business sale. While they were shopping, Sylvia left the store and found two policemen. She told them that she was a drug addict and needed help. A few hours later, she was admitted to Elmhurst. She spent a month at Elmhurst, and then, on February 6, 1976, she was transferred to Creedmoor.

Eighteen

When Sylvia Frumkin was admitted to Creedmoor for the sixth time, the Clearview unit had moved to Building N/4, which had opened in 1932. N/4's roof had started to leak in 1933, and the building had continued to age prematurely over the following decades. When Miss Frumkin was admitted, she gave her religion as Hebrew-Christian. She was preoccupied with religion, but declined to discuss her auditory religious hallucinations with the psychologist and the psychiatrist who interviewed her, because they were "too private." The diagnosis of Miss Frumkin's illness was schizophrenia, chronic undifferentiated type.

The psychiatrist who treated Miss Frumkin in the Clearview unit first prescribed a combination of Mellaril and Haldol for her. He gradually raised the dose of Haldol. On March 12, he dropped the Mellaril and raised the daily dose of Haldol to 50 milligrams — the equivalent of 2500 milligrams of Thorazine — where he kept it for the rest of March and all of April. Miss Frumkin's condition appeared to improve. In April, she attended a sheltered workshop, where she did such benchwork-assembly tasks as packaging cutlery, paper napkins, and condiments in cellophane for use by airlines. In mid-April, she was transferred to the Clearview Motivation Center, a "hotel" on the Creedmoor grounds that had opened in 1975 for patients who no longer needed to be confined in a locked ward. In May, Miss Frumkin's psychiatrist lowered her dose of Haldol to 40 milligrams. When her condition suddenly deteriorated in June, he raised it to 50 milligrams again. Her condition continued to deteriorate: A few weeks later, she had to be sent back to the ward; in July, she could no longer attend the sheltered workshop. The psychiatrist kept raising the dosage of Haldol — to 80 milligrams in late June, to 110 milligrams in July, to 150 milligrams in mid-August, to 200 milligrams at the end of August, to 250 milligrams on September 1. On this large dose of Haldol, Miss Frumkin at first showed some improvement, but by September 19 she was attacking numerous employees and was refusing to eat. On September 22, 1976, she weighed only 108 pounds — a loss of 88 pounds altogether since the summer of 1974. While it was characteristic of her to hit attendants during episodes of acute psychosis, she usually gained weight during these episodes. On September 23, Miss Frumkin was given 300 milligrams of Haldol — the equivalent of 15,000 milligrams of Thorazine. She was still experiencing delusions, hallucinations, and confusion, and had become extremely unsteady on her feet. After she had stumbled and fallen a number of times, her psychiatrist started to lower her dose of Haldol — to 200 milligrams on October 13, to 150 milligrams on October 21, to 100 milligrams on November 15. Her bad behavior continued, but she started to eat, and she gained weight rapidly. In December, another psychiatrist at Clearview looked at the record of Miss Frumkin's fifth Creedmoor hospitalization and learned that she had improved and had been discharged on 80 milligrams of Stelazine. On December 9, she was therefore switched from Haldol to 40 milligrams of Stelazine; on December 16, this rose to 60 milligrams of Stelazine; on January 13, to 80 milligrams. Her behavior improved almost as soon as she was switched to Stelazine. In January, she started to attend the Clearview Day Center. On

February 8, 1977 — a year and two days after her sixth admission to Creedmoor — she moved back into the Clearview hotel. In April of 1977, she returned to the sheltered workshop part time. She eventually dropped out of the Day Center and went to the sheltered workshop full time.

In the fall of 1976, when Miss Frumkin's condition was at its worst, she had been brought to the attention of Dr. Werner. Irving Frumkin had written to Dr. Werner about the intolerable conditions in her ward at Clearview. As a result of one of his letters, in which he wrote that he had banged on an outer door of the ward for twenty minutes before being let in, doorbells had been installed next to the ward's outer doors. Dr. Werner believed that a psychiatrist should practice his trade, and he took a few hours each week from his directorial duties to hold individual therapy sessions with a few patients. Miss Frumkin had become one of them. She saw him once a week. When Miss Frumkin told Dr. Werner that she wanted to get out of the hospital, that her parents had made it clear they did not want her to live at home, and that she wanted to try out a new program that had recently opened on the Creedmoor grounds, Dr. Werner asked the social worker at the Clearview hotel to try to get her into this program, which was called Transitional Services. The social worker didn't believe that Miss Frumkin was ready for Transitional Services but did the extensive paperwork necessary to get her discharged from Creedmoor and accepted there. Few social workers will resist a hospital director.

Harriet Frumkin was also opposed to her daughter's going to Transitional Services in the spring of 1977. She, too, didn't believe that Sylvia was ready for it. Sylvia had made weekend visits home, but they had not gone well. The progress notes that the therapy aides at the Clearview hotel wrote on Miss Frumkin frequently read as if they thought she should be sent back to the ward rather than on to Transitional Services. On May 10, 1977, one therapy aide wrote:

Patient's hygiene and cleaning of her room area are still under supervision. Her clothing and makeup are examples of her impulsive, compulsive sets of decisions, as well as her supposed diet. Examples are: Makeup heavily smeared on her face, in dining room she sneaks around and eats other pts. desserts, salad, etc. Clothing is either too tight, too short, too long, unmatched jewelry, etc. The wilder her attire, the happier she seems to be. When Sylvia is approached, she resents the fact, and generally babbles off so much. It has also been brought to my attention that Sylvia relates only to doctors and those with authority.

On June 14, 1977, Sylvia Frumkin was transferred to Transitional Services.

⸻

It is only a two-block walk along Creedmoor's Avenue A from the Clearview hotel to Building 20, a former staff residence that has been used since 1975 to house some of the clients in Phase 1 of the Transitional Services program, but it meant a great deal to Miss Frumkin to be told that she could walk those two blocks. She continued to go to the sheltered workshop, to see Dr. Werner for therapy, and to live on the grounds, in a double room, but there were differences between being at the hotel and being at Transitional that may have seemed small to some but were not so small to Miss Frumkin. At Transitional, she had a key to her room and she was permitted to call her counselors by their first names. As she got older, Miss Frumkin had come to resent the fact that some of the people with authority over her were younger than she was (it heightened her sense of time ticking away), and that she had to call them Mr. or Mrs. or Miss, while they called her Sylvia.

In Phase 1 of Transitional, clients were assigned to counselors who taught them skills they would need when they progressed, after a few months, to Phase 2 (living under close supervision in small apartments, on the grounds or in the community, where they were responsible for doing their own grocery shopping and cooking) and then to Phase 3 (living under minimal supervision in apartments in Queens that had been rented by Transitional Services). While Miss Frumkin was in Transitional, she was taught how to plan a meal, shop for its ingredients (she was unfamiliar with such concepts as unit pricing), cook the meal, and clean up afterward. Her counselors' notes indicated that she could cook quite well but didn't like to clean up and usually left the kitchen in a mess. "Instructions not needed — pushing was," one counselor wrote. Miss Frumkin, whose weight had increased a great deal in recent months, tried Weight Watchers for a brief period but got discouraged and abandoned the diet. Another counselor commented on her eating habits and tried to get a stopwatch, so that she would know just how fast she was eating.

A number of people — Joyce Frumkin is one of them — remembered that there were some days in the summer and fall of 1977 when Sylvia appeared "quite normal." Dr. Werner was another person who had that impression. In the summer of 1977, Dr. Werner decided to lower Miss Frumkin's medication. In July, he told her to skip taking her eighty milligrams of Stelazine on weekends. In August, he lowered her medication to seventy milligrams of Stelazine a day, five days a week. On October 25, he cut her Stelazine to fifty milligrams a day five days a week, and wrote in one of the reports he periodically sent to Transitional Services that she was making considerable progress "not only in living but in her ability to seek gainful employment," and that he would be gradually diminishing her Stelazine, "as Ms. Frumkin shows no sign of any serious emotional difficulties at this time." He concluded his report by saying that he hoped "she will eventually receive little or no medication." Two days later, the supervisor of the sheltered workshop wrote a note saying that Miss Frumkin was still doing excellent work. She added, "I find her extremely tense and withdrawn. Her periods of work are short and she will state that she can't concentrate and ask to leave."

Irving Frumkin came to Transitional Services to eat lunch several days a week while Sylvia was there. He also took her to Dr. Luis Santiago, a psychiatrist at a community medical center on Long Island. Dr. Santiago was testing Anafranil, a tricyclic antidepressant that is not yet commercially available in the United States. He gave Miss Frumkin an expensive series of tests — blood tests, urine tests, and hair tests. He interviewed her, and then told her father, "Mr. Frumkin, your daughter is not schizophrenic. She's compulsive." At the same time that Dr. Werner was progressively lowering Miss Frumkin's Stelazine (by January of 1978, he had it down to forty milligrams a day, five days a week), Dr. Santiago was giving her fifty milligrams of Anafranil a day and megavitamins as well. Miss Frumkin's condition began to deteriorate. Her counselors at Transitional noticed her deterioration shortly after her supervisor at the sheltered workshop had. Her room was filthy; she said she couldn't wash her clothes for a week, because she didn't have any money (she had spent it all on food); she said she could spend only ten minutes with a counselor who had planned to spend an hour with her, because she had to watch television; she kicked another client at Transitional Services and was fined ten dollars; she appeared to be preoccupied with Christianity. One day in December of 1977, a counselor at Transitional Services spoke to Miss Frumkin about her increased nervousness and changed behavior. Miss Frumkin said that she was unaware of these changes in behavior and that whatever anyone may have noticed was "nothing." The counselor had spoken to Dr. Werner, who had agreed to let Sylvia take five extra milligrams of Stelazine in the morning. Transitional Services delayed Miss Frumkin's referral to Phase 2 for a month, but Dr. Werner was eager to have her proceed. She was transferred to Phase 2 on January 30, 1978.

Miss Frumkin moved into an apartment in another building on the Creedmoor grounds. She and her new roommate shared a bedroom; they also had a living room, a bathroom, and a kitchen. They didn't get along. Although Miss Frumkin had resumed smoking in 1976, when she was in the ward at Clearview, she had given it up again in 1977, when her condition improved — and, as was her custom, she then hated it when other people smoked. Her new roommate was a chain-smoker. She fought with her roommate about smoking, but the roommate wouldn't stop, and she further angered Miss Frumkin by using the same Brillo pad to wash dishes and ashtrays. Miss Frumkin irritated her roommate by staying up until one o'clock in the morning watching the TV set in the bedroom; the roommate liked to go to bed at nine-thirty. On the evening of February 5, 1978, Miss Frumkin called her parents to tell them she was suffering from nicotine poisoning. She soon started screaming. In the early-morning hours of February 6, she was taken to Long Island Jewish-Hillside Medical Center, where she asked to be admitted, complaining that she was having extreme difficulty getting along with her new roommate, who smoked excessively. The admitting psychiatrist found her acutely psychotic. Hillside Hospital had merged with Long Island Jewish Medical Center in 1972, five years after Miss Frumkin had spent four months at Hillside. By 1978, Hillside had some locked wards as well as unlocked cottages, and most of its patients stayed only ninety days — until their insurance ran out.

⸙ ⸙ ⸙

A specialist in psychopharmacology who was familiar with Sylvia Frumkin's case history made a number of observations about the two-year period that began on February 6, 1976 (when she entered Creedmoor for the sixth time), and ended on February 6, 1978 (when she entered Hillside for the second time). "The psychiatrist who gave her Haldol at Clearview was apparently the first psychiatrist in her whole medical history who followed an essentially sound procedure in prescribing neuroleptics," he said. "I believe that when you receive a patient you choose a drug and make a commitment to it. You should stick with the drug and gradually increase the dose until one of three things occurs: one, the symptoms begin to subside; two, nothing happens, and you ought to suspect that you have one of a small minority of patients on whom some neuroleptics will not work; or, three, the side effects become intolerable. She was kept on the drug too long, and the dose was raised too high when nothing was happening and the side effects were becoming intolerable. The initial procedure was sound, but a critical error was made. It seems that no one had bothered to study her case history. One of the most striking things about Sylvia Frumkin's case history is that many psychiatrists — those she encountered, at least, and I don't think her case is uncommon in this respect — don't take the time and trouble to study case histories. No treatment she received over a period of thirteen years bore any logical relationship to a previous treatment. You get the impression that the psychiatrists pulled a drug out of a hat and gave her too little of whatever they pulled out, or that they dumped the contents of the hat out on a tray and gave her too little of several drugs. In December of 1976, she finally ran into a psychiatrist who made one of the few really intelligent moves in her case history — a psychiatrist who looked at her most recent chart, saw that she had responded well to eighty milligrams of Stelazine and had been released from Creedmoor the fifth time on that dose, and recommended it for her again. The same drug in the same dose that has worked in the past won't always work again, because we aren't the same person every day of our lives, but there's a reasonable chance that it will work, and it's worth trying. This psychiatrist could not have known that Stelazine had possibly caused the side effect of involuntary leg swinging at Gould Farm, because what had happened to Miss Frumkin at Gould Farm wasn't in her Creedmoor history. If one had known about the side effect at Gould Farm, and if one had been convinced that Stelazine had caused it, one would obviously have been wise to experiment until one found a neuroleptic that worked as well on her as Stelazine. She did not display the same side effect when Stelazine was used on her in 1976 and 1977 at Creedmoor. A neuroleptic doesn't always cause the same side effect when it is used a second time, and that may be a possible explanation. In any case, one cannot fault the Clearview psychiatrist who was conscientious enough to read her previous chart on this point.

"Had I been the psychiatrist, however, I think I would have wanted to give Miss Frumkin more than eighty milligrams of Stelazine. Her history as far back as her first hospitalizations, in 1964, indicates that she is much less responsive to drugs than most patients. Even on an optimum dose of the optimum medication, by 1976 Miss Frumkin would probably have required several months to get over a psychotic episode. The four principal symptoms of an acute psychosis are often agitation, hallucinations, delusions, and thought disorder. Neuroleptics will usually reduce the symptoms in that order. The first thing the patient will do is calm down. With higher doses or prolonged treatment, the hallucinations will go, then the delusions. What happens too often, especially when patients are drug-resistant, is that the dose is raised only enough to get rid of the agitation, the hallucinations, and possibly the delusions. The thought disorder and perhaps some delusional thinking remain. The patients are dischargeable from hospitals under current criteria, but the remaining symptoms keep them from functioning adequately on the outside and help to bring them back to the hospitals again.

"Dr. Werner should never, of course, have lowered Miss Frumkin's Stelazine, just as the psychiatrist at Gould Farm should never have lowered her medication when she was facing a crisis. For her, leaving Gould Farm and changing phases at Transitional were real periods of stress. During periods of stress, it is a serious error to reduce the medication dosage, as the patient requires additional pharmacological protection against the increased stress. Dr. Werner was seeing to it that she would eventually have to be rehospitalized even before she went to another doctor, who misdiagnosed her and put her on a tricyclic antidepressant that is often effective for obsessive-compulsives but not for the symptoms of schizophrenia. I knew and liked Bill Werner. He was a warm human being, but he suffered from an illusion common to many psychiatrists. He lowered her Stelazine for the same reason that he had the even more unrealistic idea of eventually taking her off drugs entirely. He thought that he could cure her. He was taught in medical school that schizophrenia is incurable, and he should not have forgotten that. A patient with Miss Frumkin's case history could not fail to do anything but decompensate if she was taken off drugs, and that is why Miss Frumkin has always decompensated when she stopped taking her medication herself. It always amazes me how many psychiatrists think of major mental illnesses as conditions that are curable, when most illness in our field and others is not curable. If you look at the average internist's practice, you'll see that he's dealing with such things as heart ailments, arthritis, and diabetes — all of them chronic illnesses, like schizophrenia. What you try to do with most illness is to keep it under control. You don't try to cure it, because you can't, certainly not with currently available therapies, although it is likely that someday cures will be found."

✓ ✓ ✓

Shortly after her admission to Hillside on February 6, 1978, Miss Frumkin was started on Thorazine, which was eventually raised to 2800 milligrams daily. In addition, Hillside gave her lithium (up to 900 milligrams a day) and Stelazine (up to 90 milligrams a day), but there was only minimal improvement. When tests showed elevated liver enzymes, the phenothiazines — Thorazine and Stelazine — were discontinued, and, because of her lack of improvement, so was the lithium. On April 18, Miss Frumkin was put on Moban, one of the newest of the score of neuroleptics in use in the United States, and one that had a different molecular structure from the others.

Miss Frumkin stayed psychotic during her first two months at Hillside. When Joyce Frumkin came to visit her there, she found her sitting on a mattress praying. Miss Frumkin had a weird look on her face and wore on her head a pointed cap with a tassel, which she had made herself. Other visitors remembered that she got up on tables and danced, that she broke her eyeglasses in a fit of rage, and that her speech was so pressured — so rapid and frenzied — that she would have to stop talking because she ran out of breath. In May, her hallucinations (which were primarily religious) and her bizarre behavior started to decrease. She was able to enjoy some of the many activities offered at Hillside, which has a ratio of staff to patients that is ten times as high as Creedmoor's. At the end of ninety days, however, the Hillside resident in charge of her case decided that she was not well enough to return to Transitional Services and needed continued hospitalization. She was transferred to Creedmoor. As soon as Hermine Plotnick, who has been Clearview's unit chief since 1974, saw that Miss Frumkin was back in her unit, she said, "The ninety-first day is always Creedmoor."

Miss Frumkin's seventh stay at Creedmoor lasted from May 9, 1978, to May 31, 1978. She was treated with Moban, and although it was noted that she had some religious preoccupations, she was friendly and cooperative. On May 31, she was sent back to Transitional Services, Phase 1. After her return to Transitional, she attended a program at Hillside Day Hospital. She was in a music group, an occupational-therapy group, and a women's group. She dropped out of the women's group, because, as she remembers it, she was so deeply concerned with Christianity that the things said in the group were "very offensive" to her. On June 5, a counselor at Transitional Services noted that she was pulling the hair out of the front of her head. On June 13, a counselor noted that she was unable to sleep, was up all night, and claimed she wasn't sleepy.

Shortly after midnight on June 16, she fell on the floor of the bathroom at Transitional Services and cut her head. Several hours later, she was admitted to Creedmoor for the eighth time. Shortly after noon, she was in a Clearview unit seclusion room. Two therapy aides who had known Miss Frumkin for many years walked out a back entrance to the building to go to lunch. They could hear Miss Frumkin screaming. They knew that her seventh Creedmoor hospitalization had been her shortest; they knew that the interval between her seventh and eighth Creedmoor hospitalizations had also been her shortest. They were distressed that she was back in the ward after only sixteen days.

"Is there anything to be done?" one of the women asked the other as they walked toward a nearby delicatessen.

Her companion shook her head and then said sadly, "Only in the past."

Nineteen

In February 1979, eight months after her fall and readmission, Miss Frumkin suddenly had had enough of being at Creedmoor. At three o'clock in the morning on February 7, she heard voices. One of the voices she heard was the voice of God. He told her to get out of the hospital. She got up at seven o'clock, put on the matching skirt, blouse, vest, and jacket that her parents had bought her in December, and a pair of boots and a winter coat. She crammed the fifth piece of her outfit — a pair of slacks — into her handbag and left her room at the hotel. She went to get her morning Moban tablet, but she didn't swallow it; she had stopped taking her pills a few days earlier. Then she signed out for the day. Instead of going to breakfast in the dining room near the hotel, she walked out the hospital gate closest to the hotel on Hillside Avenue and walked down Hillside Avenue a few blocks to her bank. She withdrew two hundred dollars from her account. She walked from the bank to a bus stop and took a bus and a subway into Manhattan. She got off the subway at the Times Square stop and walked to the Port Authority Bus Terminal. One Friday evening in December, when she was attending classes at the ABMJ center in Hollis, she had by chance run into Nellie and George

Klopfer on the street. They had been visiting friends who lived next door to the center. The Klopfers had told Miss Frumkin that they had left the American Board of Missions to the Jews and were now living in Middletown, a city in Orange County, New York. They were running a halfway house there and had a small church. The Klopfers had given Miss Frumkin their address and their telephone number. In the early-morning hours of February 7, Sylvia Frumkin's voices had told her to go to the Klopfers'. She went to the counter of the bus line that served Middletown, bought a one-way ticket there, and learned that the next bus left in an hour and a half. During that time, she went to a few stores in the bus terminal. She had a snack and also bought a number of items: a crochet hook and several skeins of yarn (she felt like starting an afghan); a Timex watch, which she had wanted ever since she lost her last watch, in the spring of 1978; and a large tote bag. When she got on the bus, she had a hundred dollars left. She arrived in Middletown after a pleasant two-hour ride through parts of snow-covered New Jersey and New York. The bus stopped in front of the terminal. Miss Frumkin went inside and asked for directions to the Klopfers'. She was told that they lived a short distance away, at the top of a hill. After she walked to the bottom of their hill, she was too weary to trudge any farther through the deep snow. She saw a house, rang the doorbell, and asked the woman who opened the door if she might use her phone. She called the Klopfers. George Klopfer was surprised to hear from Miss Frumkin, and even more surprised to learn where she was. He told her he would come and get her in his car; he drove her up to his house.

Miss Frumkin immediately exacted from the Klopfers a promise not to tell anyone where she was until the ninth or tenth of February, so that she would be discharged from Creedmoor. She told them that if they called her parents or anyone at the hospital, someone would come and get her and take her back to the hospital. She said she would rather die than return to Creedmoor. The Klopfers felt torn. They knew that the Frumkins would worry about Sylvia's welfare, but she seemed in better shape than she had been in late 1975 and early 1976. She said she was determined to "make it" this time. They sympathized with her wish to be out of the hospital, and agreed to take her in and not to call anyone for a couple of days. They gave her a room in their house. She gave them her remaining hundred dollars. On the night of February 9, shortly after Miss Frumkin was discharged from Creedmoor, George Klopfer called her parents to tell them she was safe and sound. When the Frumkins learned that Sylvia had been in Middletown since February 7, they were initially angry at the Klopfers for letting them worry about their daughter for two days, but they were relieved to learn that she was all right. Though the Frumkins didn't share the Klopfers' religious ideas — they were satisfied with Judaism — they thought that the Klopfers were well-meaning people, and were grateful to them for having given Sylvia a place to live after her release from Brunswick Hospital. Even if her previous stay with the Klopfers hadn't worked out, they had tried. Mrs. Frumkin disapproved of the various religious groups to which her daughter had turned, and associated some of Sylvia's psychotic episodes with her religious ideas or with what Mrs. Frumkin believed was a seeking for acceptance by a group — any group — but she said that Sylvia's mental condition was more important to her than her religion. "I'd rather have a healthy born-again-Christian daughter than a mentally ill Jewish daughter," she told her friends. She was glad that Sylvia was out of Creedmoor and out of the city.

Miss Frumkin telephoned her parents the following morning. She sounded very happy. Her father told her that he would mail her her medication. She called her parents several times over the next ten days. She said that she was going on long walks, that she was losing weight, and that she hadn't been taking her medication for a while and felt fine.

She asked her parents to mail her some winter clothes. For about a week, Miss Frumkin seemed content at the Klopfers, and made an effort to get along with them and with three troubled young men who were living with them. Miss Frumkin helped George Klopfer by doing some typing and filing for him. She went with the Klopfers to Bible classes they conducted in homes around Middletown. She ate reasonably. After a week, Miss Frumkin became less cooperative. She dieted at mealtimes but took food from the refrigerator between meals. She wouldn't clean her room. She didn't want to type or do any other work. On Saturday, February 17, when George Klopfer asked her to help cut wood for a wood stove that heated part of the house, she said she wouldn't work on the Sabbath. The Klopfers were irritated with her for claiming to be Jewish when it suited her convenience. She fluctuated so much between Christianity and Judaism that they doubted whether she was a born-again Christian. On Saturday, February 24, she again declined to work on her Sabbath. When Klopfer told her that her room was a pigpen and ordered her to clean it up immediately, she screamed at him. The Klopfers explained to her that in a small community like theirs everyone was expected to cooperate. They suggested that since she was unwilling to be cooperative she should leave on Sunday or Monday. "My voices told me when I came here I'd be with you only a short time!" she yelled. "My voices have just told me it will be even shorter than I thought. I'm leaving today." She stuffed her belongings into her tote bag. Klopfer offered to drive her to the bus terminal, but she insisted on walking. "I'm getting out of here, and I'm going by myself," she said. The Klopfers figured that Sylvia's food and telephone calls had cost them seventy-six dollars during her two-and-a-half-week stay. They gave her back twenty-four dollars. Shortly after she left, Klopfer called the Frumkins to tell them that he was sorry things had not worked out for Sylvia at his house and that she was on the bus.

The Frumkins were disappointed. Up to then, they had thought that Sylvia was doing well. They had told their friends that the fresh country air was agreeing with her and that she would stay with the Klopfers at least until spring. They had hoped that that would turn out to be true. Mrs. Frumkin asked Klopfer if the winter clothes she had mailed Sylvia had arrived. When she learned that they hadn't, she asked him to mail the box back when it came. The Frumkins then telephoned the New York City Police Department, described Sylvia, and asked the police to meet the next bus from Middletown at the Port Authority Bus Terminal. The city police notified the Port Authority police, and two Port Authority policemen met the bus. Sylvia wasn't on it. The officers questioned the bus driver, and he told them that a young woman who fitted the Frumkins' description of Sylvia had got off the bus when it stopped in Paramus, New Jersey. The Frumkins had no idea what Sylvia might be doing in New Jersey. Two days went by before they learned where she was.

Once again, Sylvia's voices had told her where to go, and once again she had kept her destination to herself. She had often listened to WWDJ, a New Jersey radio station that broadcast sermons and religious music twenty-four hours a day. One of her favorite radio ministers was Charles Rizzo. When Rizzo spoke on WWDJ, he gave a box number in Oradell, New Jersey, as his address. It was raining hard in Paramus on Saturday afternoon, but Sylvia's voices had told her to go to Rizzo, and so she set out on foot for Oradell, a mile or so away. After she had walked along a road for a while, two policemen in a car saw her and stopped. She told them that she was walking to Oradell to meet a friend; they gave her a ride to a restaurant in Oradell, where she learned that Rizzo was the pastor of the Church of the Nazarene in nearby New Milford. She called the church, and one of Rizzo's associates came to the restaurant and drove her there. When she arrived at the church, she asked Rizzo to perform a healing on her. He told her that she would have to make an appointment for that.

A member of the church drove her to Bergen Pines County Hospital, in Paramus, a general hospital with a psychiatric service. Sylvia was admitted to Bergen Pines on an emergency basis on Saturday evening. She was very excited —she later remembered that when she was introduced to Rizzo she believed he was Billy Joel, the rock singer. She told a psychiatrist at Bergen Pines that she wanted to go to the Christian Health Care Center, a private, nonprofit psychiatric hospital in Wyckoff, New Jersey, which she had often heard mentioned on WWDJ. She was permitted to telephone the Christian Health Care Center, and was told that its charge was fifty dollars a day and that it did not accept Medicaid. She decided that Bergen Pines was a good enough place to be for the time being: A psychiatrist had seen her right away; he and the many nurses on duty had been courteous to her; the food was good; and there were only four patients in a room. She refused to give the hospital her name on Saturday or Sunday. On Monday morning, when she was told that she couldn't stay at Bergen Pines, because she was not sick enough to require hospitalization, she gave a psychiatrist her name, her home address, and her psychiatric history. The psychiatrist at Bergen Pines called the chief psychiatrist in the Clearview unit at Creedmoor, who suggested that Miss Frumkin return there as a voluntary patient. She said she wouldn't go back to Creedmoor under any circumstances. She was assigned to a social worker at Bergen Pines, who telephoned her parents. The social worker told Mrs. Frumkin that her daughter had been at Bergen Pines since Saturday but could not stay there another night. She told her that the hospital would be able to keep her only until four o'clock. If the Frumkins couldn't arrange to fetch their daughter, she would be given a bus schedule and enough money to return home.

Mrs. Frumkin told the social worker that she would call

back in a few minutes. She then telephoned Hermine Plotnick. She knew that Mrs. Plotnick had two sons, and appealed to her for help "as one mother to another." She told her what had happened, and asked her to drive out to New Jersey, get Sylvia, and drive her back to Creedmoor. Mrs. Plotnick calmly explained to Mrs. Frumkin that because she was an employee of Creedmoor it would be illegal for her to drive Sylvia back to Creedmoor against Sylvia's will. "For me to bring a discharged patient back to the hospital over her objections would be a violation of her rights," Mrs. Plotnick said. "It would be like kidnapping her." Mrs. Frumkin talked on for a while about how she had no one else to turn to except Joyce. She said she knew that Joyce didn't want anything to do with Sylvia and she realized that Joyce shouldn't be involved. She then asked Mrs. Plotnick if there was any way Sylvia could be certified by two Creedmoor psychiatrists and taken back there. Mrs. Plotnick told her that no psychiatrist at Creedmoor had seen Sylvia for three weeks and that a psychiatrist at Bergen Pines, who had seen Sylvia that day, had made a judgment that she didn't require hospitalization. Mrs. Frumkin said goodbye to Mrs. Plotnick, called Joyce at work, and asked her to drive out to New Jersey, get Sylvia, and bring her home. Joyce Frumkin knew that nothing would be worse for her parents than having Sylvia at home, but she realized that at the moment there was no alternative. If she didn't go after Sylvia, her parents would, so she agreed to spare them the trip to Paramus. Mrs. Frumkin called the social worker at Bergen Pines and asked her to please have the hospital keep Sylvia until seven o'clock — the earliest that Joyce could get there. The social worker said seven o'clock would be all right. Mrs. Frumkin then spoke to Sylvia and warned her that she could stay at home only if she didn't act up. The Frumkins had given up thinking that they could ever persuade their younger daughter to live peacefully under their roof, and didn't want to go through the ordeal they knew they were about to face. They had hoped in late 1978 and early 1979 that Sylvia would return to Transitional Services or be placed in a Jewish foster home. Once she had run away from Creedmoor and then from the Klopfers, however, they felt that they had to take her in if no one else would. Mrs. Frumkin often wished that there were some place on earth for her daughter besides Creedmoor or her house.

Joyce Frumkin left her office at five o'clock, went to her garage for her car, and reached Bergen Pine County Hospital shortly after seven. Sylvia got into her sister's car warily. The first thing she told Joyce was that the Klopfers had thrown her out. A few minutes later, she said they had told her that she would have to leave if she didn't pitch in with the chores like everyone else, and she complained that they had hassled her. She then said that Bergen Pines was the kind of hospital she should have been in, that it was much nicer than Creedmoor.

"Sylvia, you've been in Gracie Square, St. Vincent's, Hillside, and Brunswick," Joyce said. "How many more nice hospitals are you going to be in?"

Sylvia looked at her sister angrily. "Don't hassle me the way the Klopfers did," she warned her sister, and she turned on the car radio. She fiddled with the dial until she got WWDJ, and then she listened to a different minister preach a hell-fire-and-damnation sermon every fifteen minutes. From time to time, she said "Amen" or "Praise the Lord" or "Hallelujah." Occasionally, she spoke out loud and laughed.

"What are you doing?" Joyce asked.

"I'm talking out loud," Sylvia answered defensively.

Joyce knew from experience that Sylvia was talking to her voices. Sylvia struck Joyce as surprisingly calm while they were driving across the George Washington Bridge, onto the Cross-Bronx Expressway, and over the Throgs Neck Bridge. As soon as they had crossed the Throgs Neck Bridge, however, Sylvia became edgy. "Are you sure you're taking me home, and not back to Creedmoor?" she asked several times.

Joyce was tempted to drive Sylvia directly to Creedmoor, in the hope that if she did her sister would be admitted, but she didn't dare. Sylvia looked at her so menacingly that Joyce was convinced she would attack her physically if they headed south on the Cross Island Parkway, toward Creedmoor, rather than west, toward Beechhurst. As Joyce reluctantly drove west, she asked Sylvia why she had run away from Creedmoor. Joyce reminded her that she hadn't been in the ward but at the hotel, which wasn't so bad, and that she had been working toward getting out.

"I just couldn't stand Creedmoor any longer," Sylvia told her. "I'm going to live at home and go to Dr. Logan Stemple, at a Christian psychotherapy center in Manhattan." She told Joyce that she had called Dr. Stemple's office from Bergen Pines. He was booked up all that week, but his secretary had made an appointment for her with one of his associates for the following morning. She said she had first heard about Dr. Stemple in 1975 and had wanted to go to him ever since, because he was a born-again-Christian psychiatrist and she was convinced that he could help her. Joyce asked her how she was going to pay Dr. Stemple. Sylvia said that Dr. Stemple accepted Medicaid, and she was going to apply for it soon after she got home. She was going to pay for her first session with his associate, a born-again-Christian psychologist who didn't take Medicaid patients, with thirty-four dollars that she had left in her savings account.

Joyce and Sylvia Frumkin arrived at their parents' home at nine-thirty. Sylvia walked into the house and greeted her parents matter-of-factly. "I've found Jesus, everything will be great, and don't ask me what happened at the Klopfers'," she said. Her mother saw her new tote bag, noticed that its zipper was broken, and asked her what the tote bag had cost. When Sylvia told her mother she had paid thirty-five dollars for it, Mrs. Frumkin observed that salesmen could always spot suckers a mile away. Sylvia had told her mother about her new Timex watch when she telephoned home from the Klopfers'. Mrs. Frumkin didn't see it on her wrist and asked where it was. They rummaged through the tote bag; they both became hysterical when they couldn't find it. Sylvia remembered that she had had her watch at Bergen Pines, and said she had probably left it at the hospital. Mrs. Frumkin said she would call the social worker there the next day. She then warned Sylvia again that she could stay home only as long as she behaved herself. Sylvia said that she would be good and that she would clean her room. She went to bed.

⸎ ⸎ ⸎

On the morning of Tuesday, February 27, Irving Frumkin drove Sylvia into Manhattan, to the Christian psychotherapy center. She found the psychologist personable, but she wanted to see Dr. Stemple. The psychologist also believed that she needed a psychiatrist, who could prescribe medication. He was able to get her an appointment with Dr. Stemple early the next week. For the next several weeks, Miss Frumkin went to see Dr. Stemple once or twice a week for forty-five minutes. She told her parents he was a wonderful doctor, because he was a good listener and because when she told him she heard voices and was in the possession of demons he didn't tell her she was crazy, as so many other psychiatrists had done. She also felt that she had a spiritual rapport with Dr. Stemple; they had both been born again, so they were "like brothers and sisters in Christ." Dr. Stemple diagnosed Miss Frumkin's illness as schizophrenia, schizo-affective type — an illness he described as a combination of schizophrenia and manic depression. (A year later, when the third edition of the American Psychiatric Association's *Diagnostic and Statistical Manual of Mental Disorders* was published, schizo-affective disorder was no longer classified as a subtype of schizophrenia. It was also the only specific type of mental disorder for which there were no criteria for diagnosis.) In Dr. Stemple's opinion, her thought process was disordered, and her mood swung from great depression to great elation. He first prescribed a small dose of Trilafon, and gradually increased it to 32 milligrams a day — roughly the equivalent of 320 milligrams of Thorazine. He told her that Trilafon was his favorite neuroleptic, because it had few side effects. He later gave her lithium, gradually raising her dose to 1800 milligrams a day. The medication didn't seem to affect Miss Frumkin, who often told her mother that she felt "as high as a kite." Mrs. Frumkin occasionally replied, "I'll have to get an anchor to use on you as ballast."

Fighting broke out in the Frumkin house the day after Sylvia came home. She didn't clean her room. Within a few days of Sylvia's return, Mrs. Frumkin was complaining to Joyce that Sylvia's room looked as if it had been in the path of a tornado. She often found herself using weather-disaster analogies to describe rooms in her house. Just before Sylvia ran away from Creedmoor in early February, she had decided that she wanted to eat fettuccine Alfredo in a certain Italian restaurant in Queens. She hadn't got around to going there before her departure for the Klopfers'. In early March, she insisted on cooking fettuccine Alfredo at home. Pieces of butter landed on the kitchen floor. Dirty plates, bowls, and pots and pans piled up in the kitchen sink. Sylvia didn't like to wash dishes. Mrs. Frumkin, who regarded the kitchen as her private preserve, told Sylvia she was too fat to be eating fettuccine Alfredo, and ordered her out of the kitchen. Sylvia ran out of the kitchen carrying a pot filled with noodles, butter, and cheese, which she hurled on the living-room floor. "My kitchen and my living room looked as if a cyclone had hit them," Mrs. Frumkin told Joyce over the telephone that evening.

During her first three weeks at home, Sylvia Frumkin spent most of her time in her room. She went out only when she had an appointment with Dr. Stemple, and she was soon canceling appointments with him at the last minute. She sat on her bed for hours at a time, her legs folded under her in the lotus position, picking at her fingernails until they bled. She often watched television until three o'clock in the morning or listened to religious radio stations, and she often telephoned the evangelists she had heard; the Frumkins' phone bill for March was sixty-five dollars. She refused to get dressed, and came to meals wearing an unbuttoned nightgown. Her father objected to her "indecent exposure." Her mother objected to the large portions of food she ate at mealtimes and to her post-midnight raids on the refrigerator, especially when Sylvia ate things that Mr. Frumkin had bought for himself — bland foods for his special diet, like sour cream, cream cheese, and coffee whitener. After a few days at home, Sylvia went on a diet. She had lost several pounds at the Klopfers', and she lost ten pounds at home while adhering more or less faithfully to a twelve-hundred-calorie-a-day diet for two weeks. During the time she was dieting, she chewed her food forty-eight times before swallowing it. "The Lord has given me such will power," she told her mother one evening. After three weeks of dieting, she weighed 170 pounds. By then, her will power had disappeared. She again began to eat great quantities of fattening foods. She stopped losing weight.

By the middle of March, Irving Frumkin had had enough of having his younger daughter at home. Her idleness, her eating habits, and her foul language exasperated him. He threatened to call the police and ask them to take her back to the hospital. "What are you going to tell the police?" Sylvia responded tauntingly. "That I don't clean my room? That I eat too much? They won't commit me for that." By the end of the month, Mr. Frumkin said he was ready to leave the house if that was the only way to get away from Sylvia.

April 2, 1979, was Harriet and Irving Frumkin's fortieth anniversary. Mrs. Frumkin recalled that on April 2, 1939, after their wedding reception in a Brooklyn catering hall, they had arranged to go by bus to Washington, D.C., for a short honeymoon, and that as they were about to board the bus she had told her husband that she would like to have some chocolate to eat on the ride. Irving Frumkin had left the bus gate and walked into the terminal. Mrs. Frumkin had thought he would return in a few minutes with a couple of Hershey bars. Ten minutes had gone by, and the bus driver had just announced that he was about to pull out, when Mrs. Frumkin saw her new husband running toward the bus carrying a package under his arm. She had persuaded the bus driver to wait for him. Irving Frumkin had jumped on the bus and handed his wife a brown paper bag. Inside she had found a one-pound box of Whitman's Sampler chocolates. Mrs. Frumkin had enjoyed the chocolates. She had also liked the festive cross-stitch design on the yellow box they came in. After the honeymoon was over and the chocolates were gone, she had kept the box. On their first wedding anniversary, Irving Frumkin had handed his wife a package, saying, "This is a remembrance." He had given her another box of Whitman's Sampler chocolates. Each year on their anniversary, Harriet Frumkin had received a box of Whitman's Sampler chocolates from her husband.

On April 2, 1979, Irving Frumkin went to the supermarket. When he returned, he put the groceries on the kitchen table. "This is the first time in forty years I haven't bought you a box of Whitman's Sampler chocolates on your anniversary," he said. "I just feel too upset with life in this house to buy one. I'm sorry."

Mrs. Frumkin told him it didn't matter. "My life is so bitter you would have had to bring me a whole candy factory to sweeten it up," she said. "I know how you feel about wanting to leave the house. If I didn't have my art students, I'd go right with you."

Joyce Frumkin had sent her parents an anniversary card and a gift. Sylvia didn't even wish them a happy anniversary.

Several days after the unhappy anniversary, Sylvia decided

that she wanted to spend a few hours each day out of the house. She received a monthly Social Security Administration (S.S.A.) disability check. She was entitled to receive an additional Supplemental Security Income payment from the federal government each month when she was out of the hospital. She told her parents she would apply for S.S.I. right away, but pointed out that it would take some time for her to receive these checks, and asked them to give her five dollars a day in the meantime, so that she would have spending money; she promised to pay them back when her S.S.I. checks came. Mrs. Frumkin gave her the money; it was worth five dollars a day to have Sylvia out of the house for a few hours. Some days, Sylvia went job hunting. Some days, she went from one McDonald's to another. McDonald's was having a Gold Rush game. To win the grand prize, contestants had to acquire four game stamps numbered 1, 2, 3, and 4. Each person who got all four stamps would receive twenty-five thousand dollars. Sylvia procured many number 1 and number 2 game stamps. At length, she got a number 3 stamp and was certain she would be a winner. She expected to get a number 4 in a few more days. For a couple of weeks, she went to various McDonald's restaurants in Queens, bought something to eat or drink, and asked for a stamp. Then she discovered that she could go into a McDonald's without buying anything and would be given a stamp if she asked for it. As she became more obsessed with winning the game, she started to go from table to table at various McDonald's restaurants asking customers if she might have their stamps. The manager of one McDonald's asked her to leave; some of the patrons had complained that she was annoying them. She left quietly. Some days, Sylvia used a good deal of her spending money for carfare to travel to McDonald's restaurants scattered all over the borough of Queens.

Other days, she spent two dollars on the round-trip subway and bus fare to Manhattan, and went to a few employment agencies. She thought that she would like to be a receptionist and that she was qualified to be one. Some days she appeared reasonably calm, and agencies sent her out on job interviews. By the time she arrived at an interview, she was invariably keyed up, talked too much and too fast, and was turned down. She started to go directly to firms that had placed ads for receptionists in the newspapers, but she was never hired. Harriet Frumkin said she hoped her daughter would get a job but didn't think she would. "You get a job? Ha!" she said as Sylvia was leaving the house one morning. "As what — fat lady in a circus?"

Joyce Frumkin came home on April 11, 1979, for the Passover holiday. Mrs. Frumkin had wanted her house tidied up for Passover. "God, your room looks as if a hurricane had hit it," she had told Sylvia on April 10. "Don't take the name of the Lord in vain!" Sylvia had shouted at her. Mrs. Frumkin had cleaned her daughter's room while Sylvia was out shopping that day. On April 11, she prepared a nice dinner. She put grape juice on the table instead of wine, because she had been told that it was inadvisable for people on antipsychotic medication to drink alcohol. When the Seder dinner was ready, Mrs. Frumkin called the family to the table. Sylvia refused to budge from the living room, where she was watching television. "I don't want to eat your lousy food," she told her mother. Over the years, Joyce had grown weary of Sylvia's behavior and of her mother's way of dealing with it. She pleaded with her mother to ignore Sylvia. Joyce was sure that Sylvia would be unable to resist the idea of everyone else's eating and would come to the table. Mrs. Frumkin didn't listen to Joyce. She begged Sylvia to join them. Sylvia finally consented. "All right, I'll eat," she said, as if she were doing her mother a favor. She ate a large amount of food with very poor table manners. Then she suddenly noticed that there was no wine on the table, and accused her parents of blasphemy. "There has to be wine; it's the blood of Christ," she said.

Joyce had had enough. She was distressed by the deterioration in her parents' health since Sylvia's homecoming: Her father's ulcers were acting up and he was losing weight, and her mother's arthritis was causing her pain. "You mean every time I have a glass of Beaujolais I'm drinking the blood of your Lord?" Joyce asked her sister. Sylvia picked up a glass of grape juice and threw it at her. Joyce ducked. The grape juice landed on the dining-room floor. "If you love Jesus so much, why don't you go off somewhere nice and far away and be a nun?" Joyce shouted. The Frumkins had purposely omitted the traditional Seder service for fear of provoking a born-again-Christian tirade from Sylvia. Now, after telling her family that their souls were damned because they hadn't found Christ, Sylvia left the table.

She stayed in her room the next morning, ate lunch alone, and left the house in the afternoon. Late that evening, she called home. She said she was down to her last dime and was in a McDonald's in Bayside, Queens, a few miles from Beechhurst. Mr. Frumkin had made numerous trips to fetch Sylvia when she called after losing her change purse or spending her last fifty cents on food. This time, Joyce went to fetch Sylvia, to save her father the trouble.

May 1, 1979, was Harriet Frumkin's seventy-first birthday. The day began with Sylvia's telling her, "You're my mother, and I'm supposed to love you more than anyone else in the world except my husband, if I had a husband, but I hate you."

"I hope I don't have another birthday," Mrs. Frumkin told Sylvia. Mrs. Frumkin said she wished she were dead almost as often as Sylvia said she wished she hadn't been born.

"So drop dead and jump into your grave," Sylvia said. "You're getting senile anyway. You've lived long enough. Go ahead and die and let me live my own life."

"I wish I could die, so I could get away from you and your big mouth," Mrs. Frumkin said. "Thank you for a lovely birthday."

Sylvia appeared to be untroubled by their conversation and soon left to apply for a job doing crocheting. That afternoon, when she returned home, still unemployed, her mother was giving an art lesson in her studio, in the attic. Sylvia decided to prepare a snack for herself. The directions on a package of frozen potato pancakes that she found in the freezer specified that they were to be heated without oil. Sylvia doused a few of the potato pancakes with oil and put them in a frying pan over a burner turned up high. A smoke detector in the kitchen went off. Mrs. Frumkin heard its screech and rushed downstairs. She took the potato pancakes off the stove, shouted at Sylvia, finished the lesson, and then cleaned up the messy stove, saying as she did so, "Methuselah was an adolescent compared to me." Sylvia didn't apologize and didn't wish her mother a happy birthday. When she went to her room that evening, she was whispering prayers; there was a slight smile on her face.

Later that evening, Irving Frumkin went for a walk. He came home carrying a package, which he gave to his wife. When she opened it, she saw that it was her wedding-anniversary box of Whitman's chocolates. "I wanted you to at least have a present on your birthday," he said. "It's been over two months since Sylvia came home. I don't know how much more of this I can take."

Mrs. Frumkin nodded in seeming agreement. "If Creedmoor weren't so horrible, I wouldn't mind sending her back there, and if she were a little crazier than she is she wouldn't mind going, but some days she's almost normal and I can't bring myself to do it."

On Sylvia's worst days, Mrs. Frumkin telephoned Dr. Stemple. He was usually with a patient, so she would leave word with the secretary that it was impossible to live with Sylvia and ask Dr. Stemple to telephone her. Dr. Stemple often didn't return Mrs. Frumkin's calls; the relatives of his other patients didn't telephone him so frequently. One day, however, he made an appointment to see the Frumkins and Joyce to discuss Sylvia. They described her behavior and asked him if he could do anything to change it. "She was psychotic when she came to me, and she's still psychotic," Dr. Stemple said. "I'm not sure if she's even taking the Trilafon, and because she's had tardive dyskinesia I don't want to increase the dose. The way she is now, she'll soon wind up in a hospital, but she's so dead set against going back to one that I'm willing to keep trying to help her." The Frumkins asked Dr. Stemple about the sessions that Sylvia had with him. "She does ninety-nine percent of the talking," Dr. Stemple told them. "She hardly ever asks me a question, and about the only time I get a word in edgewise is when she's gone on a few minutes past her session and I know my next patient is waiting. Then I finally have to interrupt her to tell her it's time to go." Dr. Stemple told the Frumkins that he thought he was helping Sylvia only because he understood the born-again-Christian terminology she used and because he sympathized with her suffering. The Frumkins left, favorably impressed by Dr. Stemple. He seemed to be a soft-spoken, well-educated man with a refined manner and good intentions.

In late April, Sylvia Frumkin had started to attend Fountain House, one of the oldest and most highly regarded rehabilitative programs for former mental patients in New York City. Fountain House, a nonprofit corporation, was started in the mid-forties, when a group of former patients from Rockland State Hospital, in Orangeburg, New York, got together to try to assist one another in making the difficult adjustment from life in the hospital to life in the community. In 1965, the organization had built a modern six-story clubhouse on West Forty-seventh Street. In 1979, many former patients were being referred to Fountain House by state hospitals and clinics, and most of those referred were quickly accepted into its day program. On any given day, about 350 members came to Fountain House between 9:00 A.M. and 4:00 P.M. and participated in meetings and performed jobs essential to the day-to-day running of the clubhouse dining room or snack bar; as cleaners or tour guides; or in the clerical unit, which took attendance, operated the switchboard, and put out a mimeographed daily newspaper, *Fountain House Today*. Hundreds of other members came to Fountain House for social activities on evenings, weekends, and holidays.

Many members who did well in the pre-vocational day program went on to the transitional-employment program after a few months. Fountain House has arrangements with about forty businesses in the New York metropolitan area — banks, advertising agencies, department stores, restaurant chains — for 140 entry-level jobs, such as merchandise ticketers, messengers, and food-counter workers. Without the vocational services provided by Fountain House, many former mental patients would remain permanently unemployed and financially dependent. It saddens the small Fountain House staff, of about sixty people, including social workers, psychologists, and rehabilitation counselors, that about twenty-five percent of the people who come to Fountain House drop out in the first week and thirty-five percent drop out within the first month.

Fountain House was one of Sylvia Frumkin's instant enthusiasms. In late April, having gone there a few times for orientation, she told her parents that it was a wonderful place. She was especially enthusiastic because twenty-five-cent sandwiches, ten-cent cups of coffee, and five-cent cups of tea were served in the dining room. She chose to work in the clerical unit. She was not interested in the day program except as a quick means to an end. She disregarded her counselor, who told her she would have to wait several months to be placed in a transitional job and perhaps longer to be placed in one of Fountain House's seventy apartments. In early May, she wrote several articles for *Fountain House Today*. In her articles, she expressed her dissatisfaction with residential programs she had previously been in, which had required shared cooking and food ("definitely not my bag"), and her longing for a Fountain House apartment, which enabled you to do your own shopping and eat what you pleased: "I'm my own person — I like to do what I want, when I want."

For about a week in early May, Miss Frumkin spoke favorably of Dr. Stemple and of Fountain House. She had given Fountain House her S.S.A. check on May 3 and had asked the membership office to give her a few dollars a day, so that her check would last her all month — a service that Fountain House provides for many members. One afternoon, Joyce Frumkin ran into Sylvia in a store between her office and Fountain House. Joyce hadn't yet eaten lunch, and invited Sylvia to join her in a coffee shop. The two sisters talked amicably about Fountain House and about Joyce's job as a divisional merchandise manager at a midtown department store. For a few hours that afternoon, Joyce understood her mother's reluctance to have Sylvia return to Creedmoor. That evening, Sylvia telephoned Joyce. She accused her of taking Cozy Carrot, an orange stuffed dog they had shared as girls, to college with her, thereby ruining her life. Sylvia then hung up.

Miss Frumkin's enthusiasms tended to wax quickly and wane even more quickly. By the second week in May, she was breaking more appointments with Dr. Stemple and had turned against Fountain House. Writing for *Fountain House Today* was a waste of her reportorial talents, she said; she wanted to write for *Glamour* instead. She complained that most of the members of Fountain House were "crazies" and "sickies." Within a few days, she was no longer writing for the Fountain House newspaper and rarely showed up at the clerical unit. She considered dropping out of Fountain House and returning to Creedmoor's typing workshop as an outpatient. She continued to go to Fountain House only to eat lunch and get her daily money and because she liked coming into Manhattan to shop.

May 5, 1979, was Sylvia Frumkin's thirty-first birthday.

Her parents, two family friends, and the Wilders — her mother's brother and his wife — gave her checks for her birthday. "I love money," she often said. "It's my favorite present." One day while she was searching her room for a book she had misplaced, she came upon a long-lost twenty-five-dollar gift certificate, which Joyce had given her the previous Chanukah. Joyce had bought the gift certificate at a department store that specialized in selling clothes to women who wore large sizes. Sylvia persuaded the store manager to give her twenty-five dollars in cash instead of twenty-five dollars' worth of clothes. (Many people who saw Sylvia Frumkin recognized that there was something different about her, and did things for her that they would not ordinarily do. She often went into a restaurant, asked for a glass of water, and got it; the next person who walked in and made such a request would be brusquely informed that the restaurant didn't give out free water, or would be charged ten cents for a paper cup.) At first, Miss Frumkin said she was going to spend her total of eighty dollars of Chanukah and birthday money on cassettes of Christian music to play on her tape recorder. She really wanted to buy makeup. She hesitated because she thought it might be too "worldly," and then announced to her parents one morning, "The Lord wants us to look good." For a week, she priced makeup at half a dozen stores. The following week, she spent over sixty-five dollars on a facial and an array of lip glosses, mascara, eye pencils, and blushes at the Face Factory, a store on East Forty-second Street that sold makeup. Sylvia whiled away hours going to elegant shops on Madison Avenue and Fifth Avenue. She admired the needlepoint kits at Erica Wilson, coveted a two-hundred-dollar pocketbook she saw at La Bagagerie, and often went into the F. A. O. Schwarz toy store. ("I wish I could live there," she told an acquaintance.) In early May, she bought a tiny, expensive papier-mâché box containing a small piece of chocolate at a chocolatier on Fifty-seventh Street for Joyce's birthday, which was at the end of September. On her shopping expeditions, she treated herself to numerous ice-cream cones from Baskin-Robbins.

Some days, Mrs. Frumkin was glad she was making the sacrifice of keeping Sylvia out of Creedmoor, and said she was learning to weather life with her exasperating daughter. She proudly told one friend that instead of cleaning Sylvia's storm-tossed room she simply kept its door closed and pretended there was one less room in the house. Mrs. Frumkin was nearly as mercurial as Sylvia. At five o'clock in the afternoon, she would tell a friend that Sylvia didn't belong in Creedmoor. At six o'clock, she would tell another friend that she didn't think she could survive another day with Sylvia in the house. In that hour, Sylvia might have thrown a plate at her (in 1979, Mrs. Frumkin had just two dinner plates left from her original set of wedding china), or might have spent an hour talking on the telephone when Mrs. Frumkin wanted to use it herself, or might have started speaking English with a heavy Russian accent and refused to stop. Some days, Sylvia came home unexpectedly early from Manhattan, and occasionally she found that her parents were out. Mrs. Frumkin spent a few hours once a week doing volunteer work at the office of a friend who worked for a national charitable organization. (She made use of the postage meter to send out some of her personal mail.) When the Frumkins were out, Sylvia had to go to a neighbor's house to await their return. She might then rage at them for not allowing "a woman of over thirty" to have a key to her own house.

Sylvia went out early on Saturday, May 12, the day before Mother's Day. She returned home that evening holding a cardboard Baskin-Robbins box in her arms. She presented the box to her mother. Mrs. Frumkin opened the box and saw a large ice-cream cake. Written on the chocolate ice cream in yellow letters were the words "Happy Birthday, Happy Anniversary, and Happy Mother's Day." Because her mother loved art, Sylvia had had Baskin-Robbins surround the words with easels, paintbrushes, and palettes in many colors of icing. Mrs. Frumkin looked at the cake Sylvia had designed. "That will feed ten people," she observed. "Why couldn't you have bought a small cake instead, and a lovely card I could have kept forever?" She asked Sylvia how much the cake had cost. When Sylvia said it had cost ten dollars, her mother said that she had spent too much money, and that she should find out why her S.S.I. checks hadn't yet started to come, so that she could start to pay back the money she owed her parents and pay for her room and board and telephone calls. The Frumkins had a refrigerator with only a small freezer compartment. As Mrs. Frumkin removed all the other things she had in the freezer, including Sylvia's birthday present to Joyce, put the cake in, and rearranged the things she had removed to make room for thc cake, she continued to complain about the amount of money that Sylvia was always wasting.

After her mother had expressed her displeasure for thirty minutes ("Joyce needs that chocolate like she needs a sick sister"), Sylvia, who had had fun designing the cake and had looked forward to giving it to her mother, looked sad. "You never appreciate anything I give you," she said. "You criticize everything I do."

"You spend too much time at Baskin-Robbins," Mrs. Frumkin answered. "Yesterday, you brought me a jar of fudge sauce from Baskin-Robbins. I'm as fond of fudge sauce as I am of arsenic."

Joyce Frumkin came home for Mother's Day. She told Mrs. Frumkin that her Mother's Day present would be a new haircut, hair coloring, and a manicure at her own hairdresser's in Manhattan on May 30, the day before Mrs. Frumkin's students were to show their work at her annual art show. Mrs. Frumkin told Joyce that her hairdresser was outrageously expensive and the trip into Manhattan was much too strenuous for her. She then agreed to go. "You only have one daughter as far as I can tell!" Sylvia shouted.

"I'm just a second-class citizen! I'm your stepchild! You never loved me!" She cursed her mother. Mrs. Frumkin replied that she wished she weren't a mother, so she wouldn't be screamed at. Sylvia went to her room and started to pack. It was raining hard. Mrs. Frumkin suggested, "Why don't you wait until the rain stops before you run away?" Sylvia settled down in her room to watch television, and stayed there until Joyce had gone.

Mrs. Frumkin told Joyce that she was tired of running after Sylvia and retrieving her possessions. She had recently sent the Klopfers a check for the money they had spent on postage to mail back the box containing Sylvia's winter clothes. She had also sent a check for postage to the social worker at Bergen Pines County Hospital, who had been kind enough to mail back the watch and several other things that Sylvia had left there. She had just spent two dollars at a shoemaker's to have the zipper on Sylvia's overpriced tote bag repaired. She also told Joyce that she had been worrying for the past few weeks about how Sylvia would behave on the day of the art show. She was afraid Sylvia would make a scene by accusing her, in front of her students and their parents, of loving her surrogate children more than she loved her, or that she would hand out born-again-Christian literature. Joyce had long since given up hope for Sylvia. Her concern was that Sylvia not continually destroy the peaceful old age that she wanted her parents, and particularly her mother, to have. Joyce asked whether her mother couldn't arrange to have one of her friends invite Sylvia out on the day of the art show. "It falls on a Thursday," Mrs. Frumkin said. "My friends will be working. You're going to be in Los Angeles. There's no one else who will take Sylvia. Your father just tunes her out. He goes to the supermarket, he takes walks, he reads his newspaper, and he talks out loud to the guests he watches on *Meet the Press* and *Face the Nation.* When we're talking and the telephone rings, he picks up the telephone and goes right on talking to me for five minutes before he says hello."

As soon as Joyce was gone, Sylvia came out of her room, threatened her mother with a bread knife, put the knife down, banged her mother's head against one of the kitchen walls a few times, and ran back to her room screaming about Jesus. "If you'd only accept Jesus, there would be peace and harmony in this house!" she shrieked. "This house is filled with evil spirits. When I go to sleep at night, I see demons."

On the morning of Monday, May 14, Sylvia got up at six-thirty and left for Manhattan. After she had gone, Mrs. Frumkin got up. Her head still ached. She went into the kitchen, where she found a note and a religious pamphlet affixed to her refrigerator with a magnet. "Please read this pamphlet," Sylvia had written. "This is the meat and drink of my Lord. It could save our relationship." Mrs. Frumkin glanced at the cover of the born-again-Christian leaflet and tore it up without reading it. She then sat down at her type-writer and wrote Sylvia a letter, which read, in part:

> Sylvia, dear, please read this & ponder. Thank you for supplying us with your meat and drink. You can have it all but please stop stuffing it down our throats. It only antagonizes us and does *nothing* to improve our relationship. I don't see where all this Jesus business has improved your rages, tantrums, foul language, and hatefulness to your own family. It made it more a travesty of love and kindness which *your* Jesus preached. "Love ye one another" — do you? If this be meat and drink for the body and soul, why do you keep on constantly stuffing and gorging your former lovely lithe graceful body and ruining and blotching up your former beautiful velvety smooth complexion. Why? You not only do not "love ye one another" but you also hate yourself. Sit down calmly and think over how you appear to others and how you abuse those who love you.

Mrs. Frumkin left the note on Sylvia's desk. When Sylvia came home, she went to her room. At dinner, she said nothing about the note. After dinner, she went back to her room, where her mother could hear her reading the Bible aloud, praying, and listening to a religious radio station hour after hour.

On Tuesday, May 15, Sylvia got up early and fought with her father over the mess she had made in the kitchen while she prepared her breakfast — an elaborate sundae, made with some Baskin-Robbins ice cream, some whipped cream she had brought home the previous day, and the jar of fudge sauce she had given her mother. When Mrs. Frumkin got up and went into Sylvia's room, she found the letter she had written to Sylvia on Monday on the bureau; she threw it away. On the morning of May 16, Sylvia had another quarrel with her father. She didn't return home until one-fifteen in the morning on May 17. Her father had gone to bed. Her mother had stayed up waiting for her. She asked Sylvia where she had been. Sylvia told her that it was none of her business but that she had been out with a group of fellow born-again Christians distributing tracts to passersby in Times Square. She said that she hoped they had converted a few lost souls to Christianity, and that it had been an exciting and joyful evening. She went right to bed.

She was up again at six-thirty. She had another fight with her father after he told her how thoughtless she had been to keep her mother up until all hours worrying about her. Sylvia left the house angrily and went to a Christian bookshop she had heard about the previous evening. When she got there, it was closed. She was supposed to be at Fountain House at nine o'clock. She arrived at ten-forty-five. She looked at her watch and saw she would have to leave immediately for an eleven-o'clock appointment with Dr. Stemple. She set off on foot for Dr. Stemple's office. She was eager to see him, in order to tell him that she had stopped taking her medication after her exhilarating evening of witnessing in Times Square. After she had walked and half run two blocks, she saw that it was already after eleven, and realized that she would be very late for her appointment. She called Dr. Stemple's office from a phone booth and told his secretary that she would be at least half an hour late. The secretary told her that Dr. Stemple had another patient at eleven-forty-five, and gave her an appointment for the next morning. Few of Dr. Stemple's patients canceled as many appointments as Sylvia Frumkin — if they had, he told her, he would not be able to pay his rent — but he had told his secretary that Sylvia was in greater distress than his other patients and that he regarded it as his Christian duty to try to help her.

Miss Frumkin walked slowly back to Fountain House to get her daily money and to eat lunch — a twenty-five-cent turkey-roll sandwich, two chocolate puddings, and three containers of chocolate milk. She started to talk about Jesus to a man and a woman who were already seated at the table where she chose to sit. The woman hurriedly excused herself. The man stayed, and told her he was also a born-again Christian. They both took out copies of the New Testament and started reading aloud. Each praised the Lord, without listening to a word the other was saying. After lunch, Miss Frumkin left Fountain House. While she was distributing leaflets the night before, she had heard about a program in the Bronx called New Life for Girls. According to her informant, a minister who was affiliated with the program also helped troubled born-again Christians find places to live. On Mother's Day, Miss Frumkin had made up her mind that she could no longer stand living at home. At Fountain House the next morning, she had been told for the fiftieth time that there was still a long waiting list for apartments. When she left Fountain House for the Bronx that Thursday afternoon, she was neatly dressed in a blouse, a skirt, and a jacket — three pieces of the five-piece outfit her parents had given her in December — but she was so excited that she was foaming at the mouth. That evening, she called her parents to tell them that she was spending the night in the Bronx with a young woman who was in the New Life for Girls program and that she had an appointment to see the minister who was affiliated with the program on the next morning.

On the morning of Friday, May 18, Miss Frumkin called Dr. Stemple's office at eleven o'clock — the time she was supposed to be there to see him — to break her appointment. He came to the telephone. She told him that she was not going to take any more medication, because she no longer needed it. He told her that it would be all right not to take the medication over the weekend, but he asked her to promise to call him on Monday morning and make an appointment to see him. "I love you as a sister in Christ," he said. "God bless you." She then took the subway from the Bronx to Manhattan and went to Fountain House to get her daily money. May 18 was Miss Frumkin's last day at Fountain House; she became one of the thirty-five percent of the participants in its programs who drop out within the first month. On Friday afternoon, she called home to tell her mother that she had not been accepted into the New Life for Girls program. The minister and his associates had been nice, she said, but they had explained to her that their program was for former alcoholics, drug addicts, and prostitutes rather than for former mental patients. She told her mother that she had six dollars and two subway tokens in her pocketbook. She said she was going to spend the six dollars on a ticket to a performance by a born-again-Christian comedian being given at eight o'clock that evening, at the Manhattan Church of the Nazarene, formerly the Lambs Club, on West Forty-fourth Street. She said that the comedian was a former pusher, pimp, and satanist priest, who had been rejuvenated since he had come into the bosom of the Lord. Mrs. Frumkin asked Sylvia what she was going to do about eating dinner, since she would have no money left after buying the ticket. "I don't have to eat," Sylvia said. "This is food and drink to me. This man is famous in born-again-Christian circles." Her mother told her not to come home too late. Sylvia said her mother shouldn't worry about her. "I won't be alone," she said. "My best friend, J.C., will be with me."

Miss Frumkin went to the Manhattan Church of the Nazarene and enjoyed the comedian's performance. Her parents waited up for her until after midnight. At twelve-thirty, Mr. Frumkin went to bed. His wife changed into her pajamas. A man sitting next to Sylvia in the audience had become quite ill during the performance; he seemed to be having seizures. Miss Frumkin asked him what was wrong. He told her that he had cirrhosis of the liver. She asked him where he lived and how he was planning to get home. He said he had a room in the Bronx and would get there by subway. She told him she would take him home. They left the church together, and she hailed a cab. The man gave the cabdriver an address in the Bronx. After he stumbled out of the cab, Miss Frumkin gave the driver her home address and rode in the cab to Queens. She rang the doorbell at one-thirty.

Mrs. Frumkin came to the door in her pajamas and slippers. She was surprised to see Sylvia on the doorstep with a stranger. Sylvia introduced the man as a cabdriver and asked her mother to pay him the $17.50 she owed him. Mrs. Frumkin asked her how she had managed to run up such a bill. Sylvia explained that on her way home she had taken a man who had cirrhosis of the liver from the church to his house in the Bronx. Mrs. Frumkin shouted at her daughter for squandering money on a man who was obviously an alcoholic. She asked her who the man was. Sylvia said she didn't know his name. "Jesus told me to take him home," she said.

"You're not the Salvation Army and you're not a missionary, and you can't be responsible for all the drunks in the world," her mother said. "You should have let him take the subway home."

Sylvia told her mother she had been afraid he would fall on the tracks, and asked her to just pay the cabdriver and be quiet. Mrs. Frumkin told the cabdriver she had very little money in the house. The driver told her she could give him a check, payable to cash. Mrs. Frumkin wrote out a check for $17.50. The driver left.

As soon as he was gone, Mrs. Frumkin went back to shouting at her daughter. "Sylvia, if you plan to stay here you'll have to change your ways," she shouted. "We don't see you for two days, then after spending your last six dollars you come home with a seventeen-dollar-and-fifty-cent bill. What kind of people are you consorting with?"

"That settles it!" Sylvia shouted back. "I'm leaving this house of perdition. Only demons live here. I disown you."

Mrs. Frumkin saw an expression of pure hatred on her daughter's face. She looked away from Sylvia's face to her legs, and said loudly, "Sylvia, your legs are bare. What happened to the two pairs of queen-sized panty hose I gave you Thursday morning? You can't run off bare-legged like this. Wait until morning."

Ignoring her mother, Sylvia ran to her room, tossed into her tote bag a radio that a family friend had given her as a belated birthday present, her tape recorder, and a few other belongings, and ran back out the front door. Mrs. Frumkin threw a coat over her pajamas and chased her daughter up the street. She called to her to come home. Sylvia was running fast. When she looked back and saw her mother pursuing her, she shouted, "Get home, you! I'm not coming back!"

Mrs. Frumkin ran after her daughter for two blocks, crying out once or twice, "Please don't make me chase after you!" After she had run for three blocks, Mrs. Frumkin fell to the pavement. She couldn't get up. "Sylvia, please help me," she called.

"You go home and Jesus will help you!" Sylvia called back, and she kept running. Mrs. Frumkin sat on the sidewalk for a few minutes and then slowly picked herself up. She could no longer even see Sylvia. It was two o'clock in the morning, and the streets in the Frumkins' quiet residential neighborhood were deserted. As she stumbled home, she didn't feel like herself. It made no sense for her to be abroad at two o'clock in the morning — she rarely ventured out of her house after eight in the evening. She had felt a peculiar sense of unreality, she told a friend the following day — as if she were taking part in a nightmare. Irving Frumkin heard his wife come back into the house. When she told him what had happened, he offered to call the police. Mrs. Frumkin said that that wouldn't help. He went back to sleep. Mrs. Frumkin lay down on the bed and cried.

⸙ ⸙ ⸙

Sylvia Frumkin ran for a while after her mother had fallen. She heard God's voice telling her to go to Long Island Jewish-Hillside Medical Center. After she had run a considerable distance, she came to a bus stop, where she knew she could catch a bus bound for L.I.J.-Hillside. She waited a long time for the bus. It was 4:45 A.M. on Saturday, May 19, when she walked into the L.I.J.-Hillside emergency room. She gave her correct name and address to a nurse, who spoke to her first; complained of suffering from tension as a result of a family argument; and told her that God had led her to Hillside. A doctor then gave her a brief physical examination and took a brief psychiatric history. Miss Frumkin told the doctor that she had been mentally ill for over fifteen years, that she had stopped taking her Trilafon and lithium three days earlier, because she had thought she could do without medication, and that she hadn't slept in three nights. The doctor's impression of her was that she was suffering from chronic schizophrenia, decompensated. He referred her to the psychiatric resident on duty, Dr. Margaret Ramirez, who agreed with his diagnosis. Dr. Ramirez found Miss Frumkin disheveled and highly agitated, with very pressured speech, loosening of associations, and auditory hallucinations; she found her to be so acutely psychotic that her judgment was severely impaired. Dr. Ramirez decided that Miss Frumkin required hospitalization in a locked ward, because she was dangerous to herself and others. At eight-thirty in the morning, Dr. Ramirez telephoned the Frumkins. Mrs. Frumkin answered the telephone. She hadn't slept all night. She had lain on her bed until eight o'clock. A student was due for an art lesson at nine, and she had just put on some clothes and makeup.

Dr. Ramirez told Mrs. Frumkin that her daughter was at L.I.J.-Hillside and that in her opinion she required hospitalization in a locked unit. Mrs. Frumkin immediately asked her to admit Sylvia to Hillside. Dr. Ramirez said she couldn't: There was a waiting list for beds in Hillside's locked units. Mrs. Frumkin begged Dr. Ramirez to let Sylvia sleep on a cot in a hospital corridor until a bed in a locked unit became available. Dr. Ramirez said that that would not be possible. When Mrs. Frumkin continued to plead with her, Dr. Ramirez said that Mrs. Frumkin had two choices. If she thought she could cope with her daughter at home, Dr. Ramirez could send her there and Mrs. Frumkin could seek treatment for her on an out-patient basis, but Dr. Ramirez advised Mrs. Frumkin against that choice. Or she could let Dr. Ramirez call Creedmoor to see if Sylvia could be transferred there. Mrs. Frumkin said she didn't think it would be wise for Sylvia to return home, because she would probably just run away again. Dr. Ramirez told Mrs. Frumkin she would telephone Creedmoor. She reached Dr. Charles Ling, the weekend on-call doctor, and he told her to send Sylvia to Building N/4, where he would screen her. Dr. Ramirez called Mrs. Frumkin to say that Sylvia would soon be taken to Creedmoor in a city ambulance. Mrs. Frumkin called the Clearview unit before Sylvia's arrival, spoke to a therapy aide she had known for years, and asked her to lock up Sylvia's watch, her tape recorder, her portable radio, her tote bag, and the good clothes she was wearing, so that they would not be stolen. The ambulance arrived at Hillside for Miss

Frumkin at nine-forty-five. Ten minutes later, she was back in Ward 043, Clearview's women's new-admissions ward, to which she had been admitted on June 16, 1978, and where she had lived until December of 1978.

According to Dr. Ling's admission note, Miss Frumkin was restless and hyperkinetic. She talked incessantly and admitted that she heard voices. The voices kept whispering to her about "God and devils." She believed that people were after her on the street. Dr. Ling's diagnostic impression was schizophrenia, chronic undifferentiated type. He justified Miss Frumkin's admission by describing her as dangerous to herself and others, and wrote that because of her acute psychotic symptoms she required skilled care and treatment in a hospital setting. Miss Frumkin did not contest the admission. She signed a voluntary-request-for-hospitalization form. Two days later, she was rescreened by Dr. Sun Ming Wong, the doctor who had admitted her on June 16, 1978, and had diagnosed her then as a manic-depressive, manic type. He gave her the same diagnosis on May 21, 1979.

Twenty

Many of the Clearview attendants who had taken care of Miss Frumkin during her eighth Creedmoor hospitalization — June 16, 1978, to February 9, 1979 — took care of her again during her ninth, which began on May 19, 1979, and continued into 1980. They had a terrible sense of déjà vu. Miss Frumkin came in as acutely psychotic in May of 1979 as she had in June of 1978, and, if anything, the course of her hospitalization was worse in the various ways by which it could be measured than it had been a year earlier.

In June of 1978, she had spent 30 hours in a locked seclusion room during her first five days back in the Clearview unit, and 100 hours during her first two weeks. In 1979, she spent 100 hours in seclusion during her first five days and 200 hours during her first two and a half weeks. She had been extremely assaultive in 1978. During the late spring and summer of 1979, she attacked more patients and was hit, bitten, and scratched to an even greater extent than she had been the previous year. Occasionally, she was bitten by one of the same patients who had bitten her in 1978: Barbara Herbert, who had been in and out of Creedmoor in 1978, was also in and out in 1979. In August of 1979, a male patient punched Miss Frumkin and broke her nose; it was the first fracture she had ever had, after fifteen years of being struck by or leaping from automobiles, and fighting in hospital wards. She was far more abusive to the hospital staff in 1979 than she had been a year earlier. She hit one therapy aide on the head with a book, bit another on the hand, and threw water at a third. She slapped an aide in the face for refusing to give her the keys to a plastic shield that protected the television set in the dayhall, and she broke another aide's eyeglasses. She spit in several employees' faces, she pulled the hair of a few therapy aides and practical nurses, and she pushed a treatment-team leader across the floor of the ward. She hit or threw shoes at attendants, dining-room employees, and cleaners, and she threw chairs at visitors. She engaged in more infantile behavior in 1979 than she had in 1978, she dressed in more fanciful costumes, she disrobed more frequently, and she applied more esoteric makeup to her face; she also ate some lipstick and said it was candy. She broke two pairs of her own eyeglasses (in 1978, she had broken only one pair), she refused more medication, and she called more black therapy aides "nigger bitches." She remained acutely psychotic for a longer time, perhaps because she was given an even smaller amount of medication. In 1978, after five weeks she got 90 milligrams of Haldol — the equivalent of 4500 milligrams of Thorazine — and that proved to be a therapeutic dose. In 1979, she was never given more than 30 milligrams of Haldol. In 1979, Dr. Sun didn't diagnose her as a manic-depressive and medicate her as a schizophrenic, as he had in 1978. This time, he diagnosed her as a manic-depressive and, after prescribing neuroleptics for her for several weeks, put her on lithium in combination with a small amount of Trilafon, as Dr. Stemple had. The lithium did not help her any more than it had in the past. The small amount of Trilafon eventually stabilized her at a marginal level. In 1978, it had taken Miss Frumkin from June 16 to July 31 to be given grounds privileges for the first time. In 1979, it took her from May 19 to August 24 to get an hour of grounds privileges.

/ / /

When Miss Frumkin returned to Creedmoor in 1979, conditions in the Clearview unit were as deplorable as they had been in 1978. The wards remained so understaffed that Hermine Plotnick did not think that Clearview met the minimum staffing ratios mandated by a district court in a celebrated case (*Wyatt* vs. *Stickney*) that had been won against the State of Alabama in the early 1970s on behalf of a retarded youth and former employees of a mental institution to which he had been committed. The Court of Appeals for the Fifth Circuit, in its opinion affirming in part the decision of the district court, had ruled that "mental patients have a constitutional right to such individual treatment as will help each of them to be cured or to improve his or her mental condition." The district court had laid down minimum staffing ratios for every 250 patients. Clearview was a 150-bed unit. Using the same formulas that the district court had employed, Mrs. Plotnick calculated that Clearview's staffing ratios were below the minimum required, and that its living conditions were also not up to those the district court had enjoined in *Wyatt* vs. *Stickney*. In 1979, the morale of the overworked and poorly paid therapy aides was as low as ever. To maintain a decent standard of living, many continued to hold second full-time jobs: Several worked at other hospitals or at nursing homes; one was the manager of a Nathan's restaurant. Some received welfare; some sold Avon cosmetics. Many had their paychecks garnisheed. The wards were still dingy; the main reaction of someone who had happened to see *One Flew Over the Cuckoo's Nest* the day before he paid a visit to Clearview was that the state mental hospital vilified in the movie was so much cleaner. Supplies were still short; periods of deafening noise and sporadic violence still alternated with periods of dullness, when shabbily dressed patients milled about idly. Most of the psychiatrists were foreigners (in 1979, more Indian psychiatrists were practicing in the United States than in India), and they still spoke to their patients across a formidable linguistic and cultural barrier. The food remained starchy. In 1979, Creedmoor spent $1.80 per patient per day for food — less than New York City paid to feed a police horse for a day. After one particularly tasteless meal, Miss Frumkin recalled that the best food she had ever eaten at Creedmoor was the TV dinners the patients were served during an employees' strike in November of 1968.

⸙ ⸙ ⸙

Soon after Sylvia Frumkin was admitted to Clearview on May 19, 1979, her parents were advised to stay home, just as they had been a year earlier. Once again, the staff didn't believe that it would be beneficial for the Frumkins to see Sylvia when she was at her worst, and they didn't think that it would be in her best interest to see her parents. Mr. Frumkin had disregarded the staff's advice in 1978, and he did so again in 1979. He came to the hospital in May and June, and was hit, ignored, and verbally abused by his daughter. One day when he visited Sylvia, she was barefoot. He asked her why she wasn't wearing shoes. She told him that she was a dancer and that dancers didn't wear shoes. She then shouted, "Get out of here, you! Leave!" After another visit, Mr. Frumkin described Sylvia to his wife as "completely deranged." Mrs. Frumkin hadn't seen Sylvia from June 11, 1978, to August 2, 1978, and she didn't see her from May 19, 1979, to September 1, 1979, although she telephoned the hospital frequently. As a result of her first phone call — the one she made on May 19, before Sylvia had been transferred to the ward from Hillside — the Clearview therapy aides had locked up Sylvia's tape recorder, her watch, and her tote bag. The radio had disappeared between the time she ran out of the house and the time she arrived at Creedmoor. The clothes she had been wearing on the seventeenth, eighteenth, and nineteenth had disappeared after she reached Creedmoor. They might have been locked up in the private-clothing room, might have been taken out of there and put in the state-clothing room by mistake, and then might have been given to another patient. In 1978, the Peruvian poncho that Sylvia had worn to the hospital on June 16 had disappeared; it showed up in tatters in the fall of 1979 in Clearview's state-clothing room, looking as if it had made the rounds of all the washing machines in every unit on the Creedmoor grounds.

On May 24, when Mr. Frumkin came to Clearview to see Sylvia and to take her belongings home, Mrs. Frumkin learned about Sylvia's missing radio and clothes. She telephoned Mrs. Plotnick for the first time since February 26, when she had called to ask for her help as one mother to another. Mrs. Frumkin was enraged. She accused Mrs. Plotnick of being personally responsible for Sylvia's missing belongings, and implied that Clearview's employees had stolen the radio and the clothes. After hearing Mrs. Frumkin out, Mrs. Plotnick quietly said that it was impossible to know even when the radio was lost: Three hours had passed between the time Sylvia ran out of the Frumkins' house on the morning of May 19 and the time she turned up in the emergency room of L.I.J.-Hillside — hours that were unaccounted for. Mrs. Plotnick said she would ask Sylvia's treatment-team leader to look for the missing skirt, blouse, and jacket. "I'm sick of this delegating, you're always delegating," Mrs. Frumkin said in a hostile tone. "I will not listen to any excuses." At Joyce Frumkin's insistence, Mrs. Frumkin telephoned Mrs. Plotnick several days later to apologize. Her apology took the form of a question and three statements. "Why did all this have to happen to us?" she asked. "We deserved better. She deserved better. Mental illness is a fate worse than death."

A friend of Mrs. Frumkin's who had heard her complain

about life with Sylvia from the day Sylvia returned from the Klopfers' to the day she ran away spoke to her on May 21. The friend said she assumed that Mrs. Frumkin must be relieved to finally have Sylvia out of the house. Mrs. Frumkin denied that she had any feeling of relief. She said that it was impossible to be happy if you had a daughter in Creedmoor — and that having a child there was worse than having a dead child. She described the early-morning hours of May 19 to her friend and told her she felt guilty for having caused such a scene after Sylvia came home with the cabdriver. "I paid the man anyway," she said. "So I should have been kinder to Sylvia. Maybe I should have said, 'Hello, darling,' and let her go to bed quietly. Maybe I should even have thanked the cabdriver for bringing her home safely, and given him a tip. I always do the wrongest things."

The friend knew that before Sylvia's departure Mrs. Frumkin had been particularly worried about how Sylvia would behave on the afternoon of Thursday, May 31, while Mrs. Frumkin's art show was in progress. She called Mrs. Frumkin that evening to ask how the show had gone. Mrs. Frumkin said that her students had all produced fine portraits, seascapes, and cityscapes, and that Joyce had helped her print up a nice souvenir program, but she also said, "Who could enjoy an art show when their daughter is locked up in a seven-by-nine-foot seclusion room with nothing but a mat on the floor?" She told her friend that if Sylvia had still been living at home on May 31 she would not have been the slightest problem. "I had figured out exactly how Sylvia would spent the day," she told her friend. "She wanted so much to see *Annie* and she loved eating out, so I had planned to give her money to see the play in the afternoon and then to eat dinner afterward." The friend didn't point out to Mrs. Frumkin that there were no afternoon performances of *Annie* on Thursdays, and she kept her thoughts to herself when Mrs. Frumkin went on to say, in a wistful tone, that the house was too quiet without Sylvia. "She was like a storm brewing," Mrs. Frumkin said. "First you see the sky darkening. Then you see bolts of lightning and hear claps of thunder. Then the rain comes down in buckets. Then the storm is over and the air is too still."

⸙ ⸙ ⸙

Sylvia Frumkin was allowed her first home visit on September 15, 1979, and went home to live on convalescent care in January of 1980. While she was home on visits and then while she was living at home, she attended the typing workshop during the day and fought with her parents in the evenings and on weekends. One evening, she prepared fettuccine Alfredo again. Her mother came into the kitchen, slipped on a piece of butter that Sylvia had dropped, cut her head on a drawer that Sylvia had left open, and had to be taken to the emergency room at Flushing Hospital for back pains. Sylvia ate constantly. By the summer of 1980, she weighed 200 pounds — an all-time high — and described herself ruefully as a balloon with arms, legs, and a head. She lost numerous possessions — library cards, wallets, all the makeup she had bought at the Face Factory, and the Timex watch she had bought on her way to the Klopfers'. In the fall of 1979, on Yom Kippur, she threw a spoonful of cream cheese at Joyce; in the spring of 1980, at Passover, she broke her mother's next-to-last wedding-china dinner plate; on Mother's Day of 1980, she threw tea bags at the walls and ceiling of the Frumkins' kitchen; on Father's Day of 1980, she ran out of a restaurant where she had eaten dinner with her parents, her sister, and two family friends, because she felt they were slighting her. In December of 1979, Sylvia had gone to live with a couple she had met who offered her a foster home. She had fought with them, and had left their house after two days. On April 1, 1980, while Sylvia was living at home in disharmony and Creedmoor was trying to place her in another foster home, a social worker at Creedmoor drew up contracts for Sylvia and the Frumkins to sign, in the hope that parents and daughter might make more of an effort to coexist if they made certain commitments in writing. Sylvia signed a contract in which she said that she would not throw glasses or dishes; that she would not hit her mother and father; that she would keep her room clean; that she would attend to her personal hygiene (bathe, wash, do her hair, dress appropriately); and that she would not eat the food intended for her father's special diet. In the contract that Harriet and Irving Frumkin signed, they agreed not to mention Sylvia's medication to her; to try to compliment her on something each day (staying in a program, attending a class, improving her personal appearance); not to chase after her when she left the house in anger; and not to discuss her weight or her eating habits. Three days after signing the contracts, Sylvia and Mrs. Frumkin told the social worker, in separate conversations, "Those contracts aren't worth the paper they're written on."

Three months after the contracts were signed, and the whole family had violated every provision of them, Sylvia Frumkin took a leave from Creedmoor's typing workshop. In July and August, she attended a summer-school bookkeeping course at Flushing High School. After completing the course, she refused to return to the typing workshop; she had again decided to sever all her connections with Creedmoor. In late August and early September, she busied herself with a new pastime: collecting coupons. She filled her room and the Frumkins' garage with coupons she had clipped from newspapers and magazines she had bought, picked up on the street, or found in trash cans. Miss Frumkin tore up all the boxes she could wheedle from neighbors or compliant strangers. She saved box tops, box bottoms, and box sides for future use. She peeled off can labels and filed candy wrappers, too, acquiring a good-sized "proof of purchase" collection for money-back offers she hoped to learn of. While she was clipping, tearing, and filing, she ate to even greater excess: Her weight went up to 205. In mid-September, Miss Frumkin returned to Fountain House. On her first day back, she told her mother how much nicer the

Fountain House clients were than the typing-workshop clients. Miss Frumkin's second set of visits to Fountain House was shorter than her first. In the summer of 1980, a doctor at Creedmoor had lowered the small amount of Trilafon she was taking with the lithium, and in early September she became increasingly violent. One day, she slapped her father. Another day, she grabbed her mother's hair, held on to it, and banged her mother's head against a wall. On September 18, Sylvia Frumkin was discharged from Creedmoor. Joyce Frumkin came home on September 20 for Yom Kippur; Sylvia pounced on her and hurt Joyce's thumb.

During the first eight and a half months of 1980, Sylvia Frumkin had apparently been content with Judaism. She had gone regularly to Jewish services at Creedmoor, and had been on friendly terms with the rabbi there. A few days after Yom Kippur, Miss Frumkin met some born-again Christians who were handing out tracts in front of a Chinese restaurant in Flushing. They invited her to drive with them to an evangelical church in Pennsylvania. She went with them, enjoyed herself, and returned to her house that night around midnight in an ugly mood. Her father was asleep. Her mother had waited up nervously for her. Sylvia called her mother a bug, threatened to swat her, and went to her room, slamming the door behind her. She stayed up all night. Harriet Frumkin lay on her bed, unable to sleep. She heard crackling sounds coming from her daughter's room, but she was too frightened to go in and see what she was doing.

Sylvia came out of her room at five o'clock on Sunday morning. Her mother saw her go into the living room and take three records from a cabinet. They were among Mrs. Frumkin's favorite records. "Those are mine!" Mrs. Frumkin shouted. "Put them down!" She succeeded in retrieving a Debussy record and a Beethoven record, but couldn't stop Sylvia from smashing a twenty-five-year-old record of "The Wizard of Oz."

When Mrs. Frumkin ventured out of her room again at eight o'clock, the door to Sylvia's room was open. She had never seen Sylvia's room quite so chaotic. During the night, Sylvia had cut up her pillowcase with a pair of scissors — she told her mother there had been demons dancing on her pillow — and had cut up most of the coupons, box parts, and cassettes in her room. She had been particularly fond of her Barry Manilow and Elton John cassettes; now she called them blasphemous. The unraveled cassettes looked like snakes on the floor of the bedroom. She had also cut down some posters she had bought to decorate her room, scratching the walls in the process. She kept talking about Jesus and demons and bugs, threatened to eradicate her parents, and shouted so loud that the Frumkins' next-door neighbors, who sympathized with the family's plight, telephoned to ask the Frumkins if they couldn't control her.

Irving Frumkin had slept through the night. The neighbors' telephone call came shortly after he had got up, and when he hung up he left the house and called the police from a nearby candy store. Two policemen came. Sylvia insisted on telephoning Dr. Stemple, whom she hadn't seen in over a year. She succeeded in reaching him at his country home, in New Jersey, and asked him about demon possession. He told her she needed to go to a hospital. She then told the policemen she would go with them after she got a pocketbook from her room. She jumped through the screen of her bedroom window and landed, uninjured, in the Frumkins' back yard. One of the policemen had been watching the bedroom door and the front door. The other had been watching the bedroom window and the door that led to the back yard. He saw Sylvia jump and land safely. He caught her before she could make another attempt to elude him.

One of the policemen, a young man, said, "My wife's a born-again Christian, but she doesn't rant and rave like this." He radioed for an ambulance.

The other policeman said, "You're cursing like this and you're talking about Jesus?"

On the evening of Sunday, September 28, 1980, Sylvia

Frumkin was admitted to Creedmoor for the tenth time. Dr. Werner, the hospital director, had died of a heart attack in 1978; his successor, Dr. Yoosuf A. Haveliwala, had reorganized the hospital so that it resembled the pre-1969 hospital. Nevertheless, Miss Frumkin was admitted to the same building that had housed her in 1978 and 1979 — Building N/4. In December of 1980, shortly before N/4 was closed down, she was transferred to I.P.C.U. 2, one of two newly created Intensive Psychiatric Care Units for long-term chronic patients. Her medication was still lithium and a small amount of Trilafon. She disliked the new unit even more than she had disliked Ward 043. Not long after her transfer to I.P.C.U. 2, she said she was still convinced that Jesus would help her — something that psychiatrists had failed time and time again to do. "Mental illness is worse than cancer," she said. "The suffering doesn't have an end point."

One man who recently visited Creedmoor sat and listened to Miss Frumkin for an hour. He later told his wife he had forgotten for a while that he was at Creedmoor and had wondered where her brilliance might have led her if her illness had not led her there.

⁊ ⁊ ⁊

It is a hot summer afternoon. Sylvia Frumkin is prancing around the dayhall. She is wearing a raspberry-colored blouse and a pair of purple slacks. A white T-shirt is tied loosely around her neck; from time to time, she pulls the T-shirt over her head and wears it as if it were a headband. Every once in a while, she takes off her blouse. She is not wearing a bra. She is not wearing shoes, either, and the soles of her feet are black. She is wearing silvery-blue eyeshadow above and below her eyes and on her lips. She is talking out loud to herself. As she roams around the dayhall, she notices three visitors — a woman and two young girls. The three visitors have come to see a patient who has gone to Building 40 for X rays. The woman and her two daughters are waiting for the patient to return. They have visited Creedmoor in the past; they know Miss Frumkin, and she knows them. She comes over to the table where they are seated, alights in a chair next to the woman, and tells her and the children that she is Wonder Woman. "You're Mary Tyler Moore," she informs the woman. "No, you're Loretta Swit and you play Hot Lips on *M*A*S*H*." She tells one of the girls that she has seen her on the Mike Douglas show. "We are all making a movie," she tells the other girl. "Creedmoor is Universal Studios. The former director, Dr. Werner, gave it to me. He gave me the whole hospital before he died. There are dandelions on the lawn. I want to pull out their roots. My skin is just like the lawn. I'm going to tear it off and pluck out the bed of dandelions. This isn't schizophrenia, it's terminal acne. My cosmetologist at the Face Factory will fix me up. Smoking doesn't cause cancer, pollution does. When I was eleven, Dustin Hoffman and I — he was the handsomest boy in the class — made up a jingle about an antacid we named Burpo Fizzo. I'll sing it for you." Approximating the tune of the old "Pepsi-Cola hits the spot" jingle, Sylvia sings:

Burpo Fizzo is a drink.
It is colored cherry pink.
You can throw it in the sink.
Burpo Fizzo.

Burpo Fizzo tastes quite nice
When you serve it over ice.
It will help, if you take it twice.
Burpo Fizzo.

As she is singing the words to the third stanza, which begins with the line "Burpo Fizzo doesn't smell," she gets stuck on the first three words of the second line. "It is said, it is said, it is said," she repeats. She pauses, completes the line with the words "to taste quite well," and then says irritably, "Oh, go to hell, Burpo Fizzo." For a minute, she looks as if she is going to cry, but she quickly brightens up, tells the children again that she is Wonder Woman, tells them that she and another classmate once composed a piece of music called "A Cantata on Beech-Nut Peppermint Gum," and starts talking quickly. "For a long time, I wanted to go on *What's My Line?* as a mental patient," she says. "Being a mental patient really is my profession. I get room and board, fringe benefits like Medicaid and Medicare, and I get paid by S.S.A. and S.S.I. But the show has gone off the air, and I may not be mentally ill anymore. Maybe I just have idiosyncrasies — you'd have to ask a doctor. And the Lord wants me to go on WWDJ's *700 Club* — that's the Mike Douglas show of born-again-Christian programs. I want to be a doctor. I want to go from the theater to the operating theater. I'm going to be a doctor or a nurse, and I'm going to have the key to my front door. Lee Harvey Oswald is a patient here. God talks to me a lot. The voice is an imp in my head. I'm a good friend of Mike Nichols and Diane von Furstenberg. I first met Geraldo Rivera when I was in Elmhurst. John Travolta's father is the Shadow. I think the Cowardly Lion was secretly married to Judy Garland. I'm going to marry Lyle Waggoner, who plays Steve Trevor. I'm going to take Lynda Carter's place on *Wonder Woman* when I marry Steve. I want to have my own show, a show called *Sylvia's.* I'm my favorite person. I only wish I could get along with everyone else as well as I get along with me. I secretly have my own show already."

Sylvia looks at the children and tells them not to doubt her, because she really *is* Wonder Woman. She reaches into a small handbag she is carrying and pulls out a piece of paper, on which she scribbles, "Muhammad Ali, apologized to me." She tells the woman that she had a large tote bag and somehow lost it. "Please go to La Bagagerie and tell the saleslady that the girl who was so nice wants to have the two-hundred-dollar bag," she says. "She'll give it to you. I told her it was worth its weight in gold. Charge it to my account." She delves into the bag again, pulls out a tube of pink lipstick that is almost used up, hands it to the younger child, and tells her, in a stage whisper, that she got it from the Queen of England. "I called Prince Charles Chuck," she says. "I'm Peppermint Patty. Charles Schulz is the headmaster of my high school. My sister, Joyce, went to college and got snooty. She left me and she took Cozy Carrot with her. Joyce throws twenty-dollar bills around at beauty parlors the way most people spend two dollars and fifty cents, but Joyce's house isn't built on rock, it's built on sand. It's a sand castle. Israel is the promised land, but New Jersey is Heaven. Please help me get into the Christian Health Care Center. I'd like to go to New Jersey, but maybe I'll go to Gould Farm. The Hare Krishnas aren't too bad, but I think they should go back to India, because they're trying to take over our country. I'm planning to go back to school to do sixth grade. I want to relive my childhood. I want to pay my parents rent, have a lock on my door, and have cooking privileges. Home is the place for me. Home is where the heart is. My father was my first dentist. I want to go back in the time machine for a while. When I was at Music and Art, I once had a best friend, Camilla Costello. She was Abbott and Costello's niece. She told me, 'Sylvia, I have many friends, but you're my best friend.' At the same time, I had a therapist named Francine Baden. Francine was my fairy godmother. Those were the best six months of my life, the only normal six months of my life, those six months with Camilla and Francine. I once told Francine Baden, 'Getting well is growing up.' I'm not sure I want to grow up. I'm going to stay Wonder Woman forever." She suddenly tells the children, who haven't made a sound, to be quiet. "Sh-h-h," she says. "Do you hear the water fountain over in the corner gurgling? Maybe I can only be Wonder Woman for two more weeks, because in two weeks that water fountain will overflow, and by then I must get out of here."

Afterword

Shortly after *Is There No Place on Earth for Me?* ran in four issues of *The New Yorker* in the spring of 1981, Sylvia Frumkin's condition improved and she returned home to live. Nothing made me happier than her reaction to what I'd written about her. "I hated to read about myself being that crazy," she told me, "but the series has made me determined to try never to get that crazy again and never to return to Creedmoor." As a result of the series, a first-rate psychiatrist in New York City has accepted her as a private patient. Sylvia recently told me that he is the best psychiatrist she has ever had. He seems to have her well stabilized on medication. She is in better shape than she has been in since I met her in 1978. When I last spoke to her, she said she was on a diet and had lost thirty pounds, and that she was hoping to move into a rent-subsidized apartment of her own.

I hope that by the time this book is published in April she will be living in that apartment and that it will please her, because I want there to be a decent place on earth for Sylvia Frumkin, my subject and my friend, and for the many thousands of other people like her.

Susan Sheehan
December 1981

ABOUT THE AUTHOR

Susan Sheehan, who won a National Mental Health Association Award for this work, is a writer on the staff of *The New Yorker* and also the author of *Ten Vietnamese, A Welfare Mother,* and *A Prison and a Prisoner.* She lives in Washington, D.C., with her husband, Neil, and their two daughters.